In a world where the sacred and the secular often seem at odds, Lee Majewski's Spirituality in Yoga emerges as a luminous guide for those seeking meaning beyond the constraints of dogma. This is not merely a book—it is a profound invitation to journey inward, to rediscover the boundless depths of human consciousness through the transformative lens of yoga. With remarkable clarity, Majewski weaves together ancient wisdom, contemporary research, and deeply personal narratives, illuminating how spirituality is not a distant ideal but a lived experience, rooted in the breath, the body, and the quiet unfolding of awareness.

At a time when traditional structures of faith are waning, this book reminds us that spirituality is not lost but evolving. Majewski masterfully bridges the chasm between science and spirit, presenting yoga not as mere physical practice but as a path to wholeness—one that integrates the mind, body, and soul in pursuit of higher consciousness. From the depths of existential crisis to the heights of personal transcendence, the stories within these pages serve as both compass and lantern, guiding us toward resilience, healing, and a deeper connection with ourselves and the world around us.

Whether you are a seasoned practitioner, a seeker yearning for wisdom, or someone simply curious about the intersection of spirituality and modern life, this book offers a sanctuary of insight and inspiration. Lee Majewski has gifted us a work of immense depth and relevance—one that speaks to the heart of our collective longing for purpose, peace, and profound inner awakening.

Richard Miller, PhD, Founder iRest Institute and developer of the Integrative Restoration – iRest Meditation Program

Spirituality has become a rare element in modern Yoga therapy as it is often mistakenly associated with religiosity. In trying to be secular, we have taken the soul out of the body. This book brings about a greater understanding of this most important part of a wholesome approach to wellness.

Every pioneer chronicled here shares life transforming lessons they have experienced in their spiritual quest. This will motivate generations to come, as they learn to holistically bridge modern science and spirituality for the betterment of humanity.

Healing is only possible when we become whole once again. Be wholesome, be one.

Dr. Ananda Balayogi Bhavanani, Yogacharya

While there are certainly upsides to the widespread dissemination of Yoga into Western cultures, the significant downside is that to increase its appeal, Yoga was shorn of much of its deep spiritual heritage. It became understood more simply as physical exercise. As a result, Spirituality is a rare element in modern Yoga and Yoga therapy.

Spirituality in Yoga: Bridging the Sacred and the Human does us a great service by reminding us of and teaching us that Yoga is actually a truly holistic integrative practice. It is a bridge to developing our own wholeness and higher consciousness, and a pathway to creating a life of purpose and well-being.

Paul J. Mills, PhD, Professor of Public Health and Family Medicine, Director of the Center of Excellence for Research and Training in Integrative Health, Former Chief of Behavioral Medicine at the University of California San Diego, author of the 2023 Gold Nautilus Book Award in Science & Cosmology, Science, Being, & Becoming: The Spiritual Lives of Scientists

✷ ✷ ✷

Spirituality, defined as a secular characteristic based on experience of contemplative states, is at the core of the historical practice of yoga. Scientific biomedical research on spirituality arising from yoga practice is growing and providing credible evidence that yoga practices can and do precipitate contemplative experiences and related increases in spirituality. This research is part of a large body of continuing research in medicine emphasizing the importance of spirituality in health, well-being, and quality of life.

This excellent book is a comprehensive and scholarly review and analysis covering the history, philosophy, sociology, science, and experience of yoga and spirituality, and is a must read for anyone interested in this important topic.

Sat Bir Singh Khalsa, PhD, Corresponding Member of the Faculty of Medicine, Harvard Medical School, Editor-in-Chief, International Journal of Yoga Therapy, *Chief Editor,* The Principles and Practice of Yoga in Health Care

Spirituality in Yoga

of related interest

Yoga Therapy as a Whole-Person Approach to Health
Lee Majewski and Ananda Balayogi Bhavanani
Foreword by Stephen (Stoma) Parker
ISBN 978 1 78775 092 0
eISBN 978 1 80501 093 7

Yoga Therapy Foundations, Tools, and Practice: A Comprehensive Textbook
Diane Finlayson and Laurie C. Hyland Robertson
Foreword by Matra Raj
ISBN 978 1 78775 414 0
eISBN 978 1 78775 415 7

Trauma-informed Yoga for Pain Management: A Practical Manual for Simple Stretching, Gentle Strengthening, and Mindful Breathing
Yael Calhoun and Mona Bingham
ISBN 978 1 83997 800 5
eISBN 978 1 83997 801 2

Restoring Prana: A Therapeutic Guide to Pranayama and Healing Through the Breath for Yoga Therapists, Yoga Teachers, and Healthcare Practitioners
Robin L. Rothenberg
Foreword by Richard Miller
Illustrated by Kirsteen Wright
ISBN 978 1 84819 401 4
eISBN 978 0 85701 357 6

SPIRITUALITY IN YOGA

Bridging the Sacred and the Human

LEE MAJEWSKI

SINGING DRAGON
LONDON AND PHILADELPHIA

First published in Great Britain in 2026 by Singing Dragon, an imprint of Jessica Kingsley Publishers
Part of John Murray Press

1

Copyright © Lee Majewski 2026

The right of Lee Majewski to be identified as the Author of the Work has been asserted by her in accordance with the Copyright, Designs and Patents Act 1988.

All rights reserved. No part of this publication may be reproduced, stored in a retrieval system, or transmitted, in any form or by any means without the prior written permission of the publisher, nor be otherwise circulated in any form of binding or cover other than that in which it is published and without a similar condition being imposed on the subsequent purchaser.

A CIP catalogue record for this title is available from the British Library and the Library of Congress

ISBN 978 1 80501 378 5
eISBN 978 1 80501 379 2

Printed and bound in the United States by Integrated Books International

Jessica Kingsley Publishers' policy is to use papers that are natural, renewable and recyclable products and made from wood grown in sustainable forests. The logging and manufacturing processes are expected to conform to the environmental regulations of the country of origin.

Singing Dragon
Carmelite House
50 Victoria Embankment
London EC4Y 0DZ

www.singingdragon.com

John Murray Press
Part of Hodder & Stoughton Limited
An Hachette UK Company

The authorised representative in the EEA is Hachette Ireland,
8 Castlecourt Centre, Dublin 15, D15 XTP3, Ireland (email: info@hbgi.ie)

For Marek

Contents

Foreword 11
Stephen (Stoma) Parker

Part 1: Awakening through Spirituality: Exploring the Evolution of Consciousness and Health

Introduction 17

1. Social Context: The Decline of Religion 21

2. Spirituality 29

3. Is Secular Spirituality Alive? 51

4. Towards the State of Yoga. 65

5. Spirituality in Classical Yogic Texts 77

6. Yoga Therapy as a Spiritual Path. 101

Part 2: From Darkness to Light: Journey of Spiritual Awakening

Introduction 149

7. Breaking Free. 153

8. The Gift of Yoga 167

9. Inner Guidance 181

10. Seeking Out 195

11. Spirituality in Action 213

    Epilogue 229

    List of Interviewees 231

Foreword

STEPHEN (STOMA) PARKER

One morning in 2012 I had come to Kaivalyadhama Yoga Institute in Lonavla, Maharashtra, India to join a board meeting of an organization seeking to certify yoga teachers. I was taking the seat of my spiritual mentor, Swami Veda Bharati, at his request. I knew a little about Kaivalyadhama and Swami Kuvalayananda's early scientific studies of yoga, but knew little of the organization or the people who were involved in it. As I walked back and forth over the next few days, I met a number of people whom I felt from the outset to be old friends, even though we had just met. Among them was Dr. Ananda Balayogi Bhavanani, whose story concludes this book, and Subodh Tiwari, Kaivalyadhama's director. At that time, Lee Majewski was a resident teacher conducting yoga retreats for cancer survivors, and we gradually began to talk in passing, over tea, and over lunch, and we discovered a common sensibility about yoga and the teaching of yoga.

Since then, we have remained in contact, most recently concerning Lee's efforts to make sure that in the rush to acceptance as a profession, yoga therapy does not lose its core advantage—a holistic spiritual perspective that goes into levels of the body–mind relationship science has only just begun to understand. In large measure this has come about as a result of gradually ending the fight between scientists and yoga practitioners over the "truth" about yoga, and the creation of a more collaborative relationship that has greatly enhanced what both yoga and science can learn and do. This began with Swami Kuvalayananda in the 1920s, and continues through efforts like those of the late psychologist Francisco Varela and his facilitation of the Mind and Life dialogues between neuroscientists and senior Tibetan monks, or Bhavanani's creation of the Institute of Salutogenesis and Complementary Medicine of the Sri Balaji Vidyapeetha of Pondicherry, India.

As a result of such efforts, the empirical study of yoga and its health benefits has ballooned in recent years, as Lee documents in the opening chapter of the book.

In the early 2000s Swami Veda Bharati, in a keynote address to the SYTAR Conference of the International Association of Yoga Therapists (IAYT), asked the participants to remember that "Yoga is not for therapy. Yoga is for liberation and therapy is a side effect." He had noticed that the field of yoga therapy had become oversubscribed to seeing people in terms of the physical body and of the medical models of disease (pathogenesis), and of health as the absence of disease. To his mind, yoga therapy was at risk of losing the spiritual depth and subtlety that makes yoga yoga.

In 2023 I received a copy of *Yoga Therapy as a Whole-Person Approach to Health* by Lee Majewski and Ananda Balayogi Bhavanani with a request from the publisher for a review. I so appreciated their effort to restore the "whole-person approach" of yoga assessment and the insistence on maintaining the spiritual core of yoga that I wrote a very detailed review, which the publisher later asked to use as a foreword for the book.

And here again, Lee has asked me to write a foreword for this new book. And again, I am happy to see her advocate for maintaining the complete depth of yoga practice at the core of this emerging profession. It is easy in the race for acceptance in the professional world to try to look as much like physicians or physical therapists as possible. I saw this happen in my own profession as a psychologist and psychotherapist. As one who had used yoga therapy informally for years with clients, I joined IAYT in 2000 with the agenda of trying to keep the psychological end of things within the scope of yoga therapy.

Thankfully all these efforts at a collaborative exploration of the therapeutic side effect of yoga practice have resulted in a more robust professional stance that has a basis in what Bhavanani has come to call salutogenesis—the creation of a state of wellness that goes beyond simply eliminating illness and becomes the basis of both prevention of illness and the ability to live creatively with illness when it becomes inevitable.

The first part of the book lays out a theoretical framework for incorporating the spirituality of yoga into the practice of yoga and yoga therapy, including explicit models for the spiritual level of assessment. As useful as this is, it is the latter part of the book that, to me, is the most engaging, narrating the stories of a diverse array of yoga therapists about the development of their awareness of the spiritual dimension of the work.

There is a value judgment often made that one should not discuss one's spiritual experiences since this runs the risk of being captured by one's ego. This is certainly a risk. But in this time, when people's awareness of spirituality and their expression of it in religious practice is at a low ebb, the inspiration and the example such stories might provide is certainly worth that risk. So I was more than happy to contribute. It is a genuine joy and comfort to know that my story is in good and loving hands. I wish the reader the same joy and comfort, and a flash of awareness!

FOREWORD

PART 1

AWAKENING THROUGH SPIRITUALITY

Exploring the Evolution of Consciousness and Health

Introduction

In an age where traditional religious frameworks are fading yet the hunger for meaning persists, this book emerges as a beacon for those navigating the complexities of modern existence. This work is not merely a collection of stories or theories; it is a tapestry woven from the threads of personal transformation, ancient wisdom, and the universal quest for connection.

THE CRISIS OF MEANING IN A SECULAR WORLD

The opening chapters of this book ground us in a stark reality: Western societies are undergoing an unprecedented decline in religious affiliation. Surveys reveal that nearly 30 percent of Americans now identify as religiously unaffiliated, while church membership has plummeted to 47 percent—a seismic shift from the 70 percent stability seen just decades ago.[1] This secularization, while liberating for some, has left many adrift in a sea of existential questions. As Walter Lippmann, an American writer, reporter, and political commentator, observed nearly a century ago, modernity's wealth and autonomy often fail to answer life's deepest inquiries: Why are we here? What gives our struggles purpose?

Yet, as traditional structures wane, we are seeing a new kind of spirituality—one that transcends dogma and thrives in the intimate spaces of personal experience. Drawing on thinkers like Jim Marion and Richard Rohr, this book explores how human consciousness is evolving. Marion's nine stages of consciousness and Rohr's developmental spirituality map a path from ego-driven existence to transcendent unity, where spirituality becomes less about external rituals and more about inner awakening.

---

1   Jones, J.M. (2021) "US church membership falls below majority for first time." Gallup, March 29. https://news.gallup.com/poll/341963/church-membership-falls-below-majority-first-time.aspx; see also www.prri.org/research/census-2023-american-religion

At the heart of this transformation lies yoga—not merely as physical exercise, but as a holistic practice that integrates body, mind, and spirit. It offers a road map to the evolution of one's consciousness, resulting in a joyful and purposeful life. As the book's second part shifts from theory to lived reality, it shares raw, deeply personal narratives of individuals who found liberation through yoga. These stories, gathered from diverse corners of the globe, reveal common themes of the evolution of human consciousness through yoga.

STRUCTURE AND VISION

The book is divided into the following:

- *Context:* The decline of organized religion and the rise of a spirituality rooted in personal experience is examined, informed by recent extensive research and frameworks such as the Consensus Conference's secular definition of spirituality (Chapter 1).

- *Role of spirituality in health:* Recent extensive research outlining the importance of a spiritual component in the healing process of physical and mental disorders is highlighted, showing that even healthcare professionals and scientists are making peace with the concept and significance of secular spirituality (Chapters 2, 3, and 4).

- *Road map to higher consciousness:* Traditional yogic texts—Patanjali's *Yoga Sutras* and the *Hathapradipika*—are examined as a way to a more wholistic and happier life. With spirituality at the core of these texts, we can evolve our consciousness and transform any suffering—physical, mental, emotional, and/or spiritual (Chapter 5).

- *Stories of awakening:* Struggle and transcendence are chronicled, grouped into themes, such as liberation (Chapter 7), healing (Chapter 8), and mystical guidance (Chapter 9). Each narrative is a testament to yoga's role in fostering resilience, compassion, and self-realization, resulting in a purposeful and joyful life.

- *Integration:* How these journeys ripple outward is explored, transforming relationships, communities, and professional practices, from yoga therapy to palliative care (Chapters 6, 10 and 11).

WHY THIS BOOK MATTERS NOW

In a world grappling with loneliness, polarization, and ecological crises, *Spirituality in Yoga* argues that spirituality is not a relic of the past but a vital compass for the future. The stories and insights challenge the false divide between science and spirit, showing how yoga and meditation cultivate both personal well-being and collective empathy.

As you turn these pages, you will encounter not just theories or anecdotes, but also a mirror reflecting your own potential for growth. Whether you are a skeptic, a seeker, or a seasoned practitioner, this book invites you to explore a simple truth. As Eckhart Tolle says: "The journey from darkness to light begins not in temples or textbooks, but within the inner silence of the meditative spaces of your heart."

Let this book guide you—not as dogma, but as lanterns illuminating the path to your truest self.

CHAPTER 1

Social Context: The Decline of Religion

The destiny of humans is to awaken, and suffering is the spiritual teacher.
                                                    ECKHART TOLLE (1948–)

The Industrial Revolution marked a significant turning point in the relationship between science and religion. As science began to focus on the material world—what could be observed, measured, and understood objectively—the role of religion shifted. Religion, once intertwined with explanations of the physical world, became more concerned with the intangible aspects of human life: morality, values, and spirituality. This division between the material and the spiritual remained relatively stable until the mid-20th century.

In Western countries, surveys have shown that since the 1950s, each generation has become progressively less religious than the one before. This trend is not only reflected in declining rates of church attendance, but also in a reduction of religious socialization within families. As Christel Gärtner notes,[1] this shift is becoming more pronounced with each passing decade.

In the last two decades, data from the World Values Survey[2] has highlighted a growing trend: high-income countries are increasingly characterized by declining religiosity and a rise in atheism. Of the 60 countries surveyed, nations such as Australia, France, Japan, and the UK, and those in North America and Scandinavia, now rank among the least religious, with these countries occupying 15 of the bottom spots on the list of "Least Religious Countries" worldwide.

---

1 Gärtner, C. (2023) "Why has every postwar generation since the 1950s become less religious?" The Well, Big Think, April 14. https://bigthink.com/the-well/postwar-generations-less-religious
2 Inglehart, R. F. (2021) *Religion's Sudden Decline: What's Causing it, and What Comes Next?* Oxford: Oxford University Press. https://global.oup.com/academic/product/religions-sudden-decline-9780197547052?cc=us&lang=en&

The United States presents an interesting case. For much of its history, the USA was an outlier among developed nations due to its high levels of religiosity, although there has been a dramatic shift—from 1990 onwards there has been a noticeable decline in religious affiliation, with this decline accelerating sharply around 2007. In 1990, less than 10 percent of Americans reported "no religious affiliation," according to the General Social Survey.[3] By 2024, that number had surged to nearly 30 percent.

Similarly, data from Gallup shows that between 1940 and 2000, church membership in the US remained steady, at around 70 percent. But as the new millennium unfolded, this number plummeted—by 2020, membership in churches, synagogues, or mosques had fallen to just 47 percent. The US now ranks fifth globally for the fastest decline in practicing religious individuals, and it appears that science, reason, and skepticism have played significant roles in this rapid secularization.[4]

The secularization of Western societies may seem inevitable, but it comes with emotional consequences for many individuals. There is a growing sense of loss—a loss not only of faith, but also of community. This void may be what is contributing to the widespread loneliness reported by many today.

Walter Lippmann identified this existential problem as far back as 1929: "Men have been deprived of their sense of certainty as to why they were born, why they must work, whom they must love, what they must honor."[5] Although modern society offers wealth, technology, and autonomy, for many, these things cannot fill the spiritual void left by declining faith. The question then arises: Is spirituality truly fading from our lives? Or are we seeing a new kind of spirituality?

A NEW KIND OF SPIRITUALITY?

One perspective comes from American mystic and author Jim Marion. In his books *Putting on the Mind of Christ*[6] and *The Death of the Mythic God*,[7] Marion suggests that traditional spirituality may indeed be ending, but that doesn't mean spirituality

---

3   General Social Survey (GSS) Data Explorer: https://gssdataexplorer.norc.org
4   Jones, J. M. (2021) "US church membership falls below majority for first time." Gallup, March 29. https://news.gallup.com/poll/341963/church-membership-falls-below-majority-first-time.aspx
5   Arnold-Forster, T. (2023) "Walter Lippmann and public opinion." *American Journalism* 40, 1, 51–79. www.tandfonline.com/doi/full/10.1080/08821127.2022.2161665
6   Marion, J. (2000) *Putting on the Mind of Christ: The Inner Work of Christian Spirituality*. Charlottesville, VA: Hampton Roads Publishing Company, Inc.
7   Marion, J. (2004) *The Death of the Mythic God: The Rise of Evolutionary Spirituality*. Charlottesville, VA: Hampton Roads Publishing Company, Inc.

itself is disappearing. Instead, he argues that we are witnessing the death of what he calls "the mythic God." This God was patriarchal and legalistic—a deity who required obedience to laws but offered salvation through external rituals. Because the mythic God was a separate being, he required that we pray to him for our needs, and did not require much responsibility from an individual because they were saved in any case by adherence to the law. The church or temple guided people to God through the observance of external things such as sacraments, rituals, pilgrimages, and moral laws.

Marion proposes that we are entering what in Christianity Jesus prophesied as "the Age of Spirit." In this new era, people will no longer worship God through external means, but will instead seek God "in spirit and truth." This shift represents a move toward mysticism—where God is experienced as an experiential inner reality.

In fact, a mystical experience can be defined as transformation from the feeling of being a separate, isolated self to the sensation of being completely interconnected with the universe. This evolution in (non)self-awareness goes by many names: *samadhi*, *moksha*, unity consciousness, and Christ consciousness, among others. Such mystical experience can be encountered only within our own being after transcending ego. We need to die first to our ego, that is, to die to the separate sense of self, in order to experience this reality.

Today millions are exploring spirituality outside traditional religious frameworks. Marion believes that this signals an evolution in human consciousness—a process that continues beyond homo sapiens as we know them. The human consciousness continues to evolve at both individual and social or collective levels.

Marion outlines nine levels of consciousness through which individuals evolve:[8]

1. *Archaic consciousness*, seen in infants
2. *Magical consciousness*, present in young children
3. *Mythic consciousness*, common among pre-adolescents
4. *Rational consciousness*, typical for teenagers and adults
5. *Vision-logic consciousness*, found among pioneers at the cutting edge of consciousness today
6. *Psychic consciousness*, experienced by beginning contemplatives
7. *Subtle consciousness*, attained by advanced contemplatives and mystics

---

8   Marion, J. (2004) *The Death of the Mythic God: The Rise of Evolutionary Spirituality*. Charlottesville, VA: Hampton Roads Publishing Company, Inc.

8. *Christ or casual consciousness*, reached by those who follow Jesus or another deity deeply
9. *Nondual consciousness*, where one identifies fully with God.

People at each level of consciousness have their own worldviews. They see and understand the world in a different way from people at other levels. Their values are different, their concept of God is different, and their behavior, too, is often different. Moreover, as our consciousness evolves, we become less and less egocentric and more and more universally compassionate.

Another framework for understanding spiritual development comes from contemporary mystic Richard Rohr, a Franciscan friar. He offers his own basic overview of the stages of spiritual development, which also account for our developmentally appropriate psychological needs:[9]

1. *My body and self-image are who I am:* We focus on our own security, safety, and defense needs.

2. *My external behavior is who I am:* We need to look good from the outside and to hide any "contrary evidence" from others, and eventually from ourselves. The ego's "shadow" begins to emerge.

3. *My thoughts and feelings are who I am:* We begin to take pride in our "better" thoughts and feelings and learn to control them, so much so that we do not even see their self-serving nature. For nearly all of us, a major defeat, shock, or humiliation must be suffered and passed through to go beyond this stage.

4. *My deeper intuitions are who I am:* This is such a breakthrough and so helpful that many of us are content to stay here, but to remain at this level may lead to inner work or body work as a substitute for any real encounter with, or sacrifice for, the "other."

5. *My shadow self is who I am:* This is the first "dark night of the senses"—when our weakness overwhelms us, and we finally face ourselves in our unvarnished and uncivilized state. Without guidance, grace, and prayer, most of us go running back to previous identities.

---

9   Rohr, R. (2024) "A maturing spirituality." Daily Meditations, Center for Action and Contemplation, June 17. https://cac.org/daily-meditations/a-maturing-spirituality

6. *I am empty and powerless:* Some call this sitting in "God's waiting room," but it is more often known as "the dark night of the soul." At this point, almost any attempt to save ourselves by any superior behavior, morality, or prayer technique will fail us. All we can do is to ask, wait, and trust. God is about to become real. The false or separate self is dying in a major way.

7. *I am more than I thought I was:* We experience the permanent waning of the false self and the ascent of the True Self as the center of our being. It feels like an absence or void, even if a wonderful void. John of the Cross calls this "luminous darkness." We grow not by knowing or understanding, but only by loving and trusting.

8. *The Father and I are one:* Here, there is only God. There is nothing we need to protect, promote, or prove to anyone, especially ourselves. Our false self no longer guides the ship. We have learned to let Grace and Mystery guide us—still without full (if any) comprehension (see John 10:30).

9. *I am who I am:* I'm "just me," warts and all. We are now fully detached from our own self-image and living in God's image of us—which includes and loves both the good and the bad. We experience true serenity and freedom. This is the peace of full resting in God, the world cannot give (see John 14:27).

Rohr's stages correspond closely with Marion's levels—both suggest that most people today are somewhere between stages 3 and 4 (mythic/rational consciousness), identifying with their body, the image of their body, or thoughts/emotions. However, a growing number are reaching higher levels through spiritual practices such as yoga or meditation.

I particularly like the metaphor American mystic Caroline Myss[10] uses, describing a person represented by a nine-story building. Each story represents a certain level of consciousness, with corresponding values and ways of seeing the world. When we perceive the world from the first floor, our perspective is very limited. We see the trash and smell the dirt on the street, and hear the noise of the traffic. There seems to be limited possibility for seeing any beauty in the world. But when we take the elevator to the penthouse, our perspective is suddenly completely different. We do not see or smell the trash or hear the noise of the traffic. The view

---

10 See www.myss.com

is wide and far into the horizon, and full of beautiful vistas all around. And when we see the city in the night, it is stunningly gorgeous; we may even see some stars, too. Our whole reality is completely transformed.

To the point Marion makes—people living on each floor then have a particular perspective of seeing the world that represents a certain point of view and values. People living on the lower floors have no knowledge and understanding of the perspective and values of those who live on the higher floors. However, those who live on the higher floors understand the reality and perspective of those living on the lower floors because most of them have lived there too, before moving up. And to move up, they had to do their inner work to expand their consciousness and transcend their self/ego,[11] to see the world from a higher floor, which, in turn, transformed their reality. In addition, the lower floors are filled with multitudes of people. But as people move up the floors, the amount of people becomes reduced to only a few people "living" at the penthouse level.

Ken Wilber calls such gradual expansion of consciousness "Waking Up" in his Special Commentary in Paul Mills' book.[12] "Waking Up" refers to the overall process of transcendence of conventional self/ego and moving up the Marion scale. Wilber distinguishes this from "Growing Up," which refers to the specific stages that the self/ego goes through, as it grows and evolves in the conventional world. This "Growing Up" is closer to Rohr's framework of appropriate developmental psychological needs.

Why is it important to understand this distinction? Because no matter what state of "Waking Up" (consciousness) the person is at, they will interpret that state using the stage of "Growing Up" (psychological maturity) they are in. This explains why there are different levels of perceived reality, values, and perspectives at each floor of Myss's metaphorical building. It also clarifies why the "Growing Up" stage is a limiting factor in understanding higher floor reality.

While traditional forms of religion may be fading in many parts of the world—particularly in Western societies—spirituality itself is evolving into new forms that emphasize personal experience over religious institutional dogma. It is important therefore to bring back the role of spirituality to our everyday conversations. I only hope that this book will spark more discussions around the dinner table and in social circles.

---

11 I have used "self" to mean ego, and "Self" meaning the Divinity within each of us.
12 Wilber, K. (2022) "Special Commentary: Recognizing and Evolving Our Spiritual and Human Natures." In P. J. Mills (Ed.) *Science, Being, & Becoming: The Spiritual Lives of Scientists* (pp.ix–xvi). Fort Lauderdale, FL: Light on Light Press.

FILLING THE VOID: SPIRITUALITY IN SECULAR SOCIETY

The decline of religious affiliation has left many individuals grappling with a sense of loss—loss of community, purpose, and connection to something greater than themselves. As surveys and studies have shown, this decline is not just about fewer people attending church or following traditional religious practices; it also reflects a broader disengagement from spiritual values that once shaped human interactions and societal norms.

Although the secularization of society has brought about many advances in science, technology, and individual autonomy, as Walter Lippmann pointed out nearly a century ago, modern life often leaves people feeling deprived of meaning. Without a sense of purpose or connection to something transcendent, many struggle with the existential questions: Why are we here? What is the point of our work? Where do we turn in times of sorrow or defeat? These are questions that neither wealth nor technology can answer.

By reintroducing spirituality into our conversations—whether through discussions on deeper existential questions, purpose, or personal growth—we can begin to fill this void. Spirituality does not necessarily have to be tied to organized religion; rather, it can be about fostering deeper connections with ourselves and others. It can help us navigate the complexities of modern life by offering a framework for understanding our place in the world and the values that guide us.

One of the most significant consequences of declining religiosity is the erosion of community bonds. For centuries, religious institutions provided not only spiritual guidance but also social cohesion. Churches, mosques, temples, and synagogues were places where people gathered to support one another through life's challenges. As these institutions lose their influence, many individuals find themselves isolated and lonely. Bringing spirituality back into everyday conversations can help rebuild these connections. When we engage in discussions about the meaning of life, compassion, and shared values, we create spaces where people feel heard and understood. These conversations foster empathy and mutual respect—qualities that are essential for building strong communities in an increasingly fragmented world.

Spirituality also plays a key role in personal development. As Marion suggests in his exploration of consciousness levels, true spiritual growth comes from within—it is an experiential reality that transcends ego and connects us to something greater than ourselves. By incorporating spirituality into our daily lives, we open ourselves up to deeper self-awareness and inner peace. Incorporating spiritual practices such as prayer, meditation, and mindfulness, or simply reflecting on our values can lead to profound personal transformation. These practices help us cultivate qualities such as patience, gratitude, and compassion—traits that not only enhance our own well-being, but also improve our relationships with others.

The modern world presents us with unprecedented challenges—environmental crises, political polarization, mental health struggles—that require more than just technical solutions. Spirituality offers a way to approach these issues with a sense of purpose and interconnectedness. When we view the world through a spiritual lens, we recognize that we are all part of a larger whole. This perspective encourages us to act with greater responsibility toward others and the planet.

As society continues to evolve away from traditional religious frameworks, it is essential that we find new ways to integrate spirituality into our daily lives. This does not mean returning to dogmatic practices or rigid belief systems; rather, it means fostering open conversations about meaning, purpose, and values that transcend material concerns. By bringing spirituality back into everyday conversations—whether through discussions on mindfulness practices or reflections on personal growth—we can help fill the void left by secularization. In doing so, we create opportunities for deeper connection with ourselves and others while navigating the complexities of modern life with greater clarity and compassion.

Ultimately, spirituality offers a path toward healing, both individually and collectively—a path that leads not only to personal fulfillment but also to stronger communities built on shared values of empathy and mutual respect. I do hope that this book will help to break the silence and inspire discussions on spirituality in our everyday conversations.

CHAPTER 2

Spirituality

Freedom is not the capacity to be what we are not, but the capacity to be fully who we already are, to develop our inherent selves as much as divine time and circumstances allow.

RICHARD ROHR (1943–)[1]

EVOLUTION OF DEFINITION

With religiosity in decline in the Western world, a parallel phenomenon emerged toward the end of the 20th century—spirituality. In 1997 Kendler and colleagues published groundbreaking research suggesting that spirituality wasn't merely a belief system imposed from the outside but rather an innate capacity that each of us was born with.[2] Kendler's team also highlighted the protective psychological benefits of spirituality, especially during times of stress, illness, or loss. This revelation opened the door to a broader, more inclusive understanding of spirituality, distinct from traditional religious beliefs.

Interest in spirituality grew exponentially after 2000, but with this came a certain level of perplexity as the word seemed to mean different things for different people. Researchers also struggled to define "spirituality," with many early studies using the term interchangeably with religion. For example, in 1990, Vanderpool and Levin wrote that "through medicine and religion, humans grapple with common issues of infirmity, suffering, loneliness, despair, and death, while searching for hope, meaning, and personal value in the crisis of

---

1 Rohr, R. ([1996] 2022) *Jesus' Alternative Plan: The Sermon on the Mount, 2nd edn.* Cincinnati, OH: Franciscan Media, pp.14–16.
2 Kendler, K. S., Gardner, C. O., and Prescott, C. A. (1997) "Religion, psychopathology, and substance use and abuse: A multimeasure, genetic-epidemiologic study." *American Journal of Psychiatry 154,* 322–329. https://doi.org/10.1176/ajp.154.3.322

illness."[3] However, by 2006, MacKinlay offered a more individualized definition: "Spirituality is an individual's attempt to find meaning and purpose in life."[4] Two years later, Wiklund expanded on this definition by adding the idea of relationships—among human beings, nature, and the divine.[5]

This confusion over definitions led to the Consensus Conference in 2009 in Pasadena, California, the first of many such gatherings. The conference brought together healthcare professionals and spiritual leaders who believed that spiritual care was a fundamental component of quality palliative care. Through a collaborative process, they developed a broad and inclusive definition of spirituality: "Spirituality is the aspect of humanity that refers to the way individuals seek and express meaning and purpose, and the way they experience their connectedness to the moment, to self, to others, to nature, and to the significant or sacred."[6]

This definition marked a significant turning point. It secularized spirituality and applied it to everyone—religious, atheist, agnostic, or otherwise. As a result, spirituality could now be researched and discussed in scientific contexts, particularly in relation to health, without encroaching on the domain of religion. Unsurprisingly, the number of research papers on spirituality exploded. Between 2010 and early 2024, PubMed listed over 19,000 studies on spirituality, most published in medical journals.

The definition proposed by the Consensus Conference was widely accepted as a starting point, but not as a final definition. The interest within the research community forged widespread discussions within healthcare, and the definition kept evolving according to the specific needs of the community. In 2011, the European Association of Palliative Care (EAPC) proposed a slightly different take: "Spirituality is the dynamic dimension of human life that relates to the way persons (individual and community) experience, express and/or seek meaning, purpose and transcendence, and the way they connect to the moment, to self, to others, to nature, to the significant and/or the sacred."[7]

---

3   Vanderpool, H. Y. and Levin, J. S. (1990) "Religion and medicine: How are they related?" *Journal of Religion and Health 29*, 1, 9–20. doi: 10.1007/BF00987090.
4   MacKinlay, E. (2006) "Spiritual care: Recognizing spiritual needs of older adults." *Journal of Religion, Spirituality & Aging 18*, 2–3, 59–71. https://doi.org/10.1300/J496v18n02_05
5   Wiklund, L. (2008) "Existential aspects of living with addiction: Part II: Caring needs. A hermeneutic expansion of qualitative findings." *Journal of Clinical Nursing 17*, 18, 2435–2443. https://doi.org/10.1111/j.1365-2702.2008.02357.x
6   Puchalski, C. M., Ferrell, B., Virani, R., Otis-Green, S., *et al.* (2009) "Improving the quality of spiritual care as a dimension of palliative care: The report of the Consensus Conference." *Journal of Palliative Medicine 12*, 10, 885–904. doi: 10.1089/jpm.2009.0142.
7   https://eapcnet.eu/eapc-groups/reference/spiritual-care

In 2018, the US Veteran Association Handbook proposed:[8]

Spirituality is our experience of how we relate to whatever is greater than ourselves and gives meaning to our lives… At the same time, it also involves how we are connected to one another.

- Connection to a higher power
- Connection to humankind
- Connection to nature
- Connection to oneself.

In 2014 GWish (GW Institute for Spirituality & Health), established in 2001 within the George Washington University School of Medicine and Health Sciences, further developed the Consensus Conference's 2009 definition, secularizing it, and formulating four domains:[9]

Spirituality is a dynamic and intrinsic aspect of humanity through which persons seek ultimate meaning, purpose and transcendence, and experience relationship to self, family, others, community, society, nature, and the significant or sacred. Spirituality is expressed through beliefs, values, traditions and practices.

Spirituality can be seen in four domains:

- *Qualities of being*—love, hope, meaning, and purpose, transcendent identity, intrinsic value, and dignity of the person
- *Spiritual values* that have an impact on coping and on healthcare decisions
- *Relationship or connection* to a transcendent power (vertical connection to something greater) and to other people (horizontal connection)
- *Spiritual practices* that nurture the person and enhance wellness (rituals, sacraments, prayers, meditation, etc.).

These are only a few examples of the many definitions of spirituality. Many researchers have struggled with the definition of spirituality and proposed some kind of variant or focused on only one dimension. Finally, de Brito Sena, with colleagues, reviewed 166 definitions of spirituality published in scientific journals

---

[8] www.va.gov/WHOLEHEALTH/Veteran-Handouts/docs/IntroSpiritSoul-508Final-9-5-2018.pdf
[9] Puchalski, C. M., Ferrell, B., Virani, R., Otis-Green, S., *et al.* (2009) "Improving the quality of spiritual care as a dimension of palliative care: The report of the Consensus Conference." *Journal of Palliative Medicine 12*, 10, 885–904. doi: 10.1089/jpm.2009.0142.

up to 2020. Theirs was the first study to systematically evaluate the most important and highly cited spirituality definitions under the healthcare field instead of focusing on one specific population, such as nursing or palliative care. Their research outcome, published in *Frontiers of Psychology*,[10] proposed a framework, enabling flows (how they read the chart) according to the individual's context and experience, and allowing for distinct cultural, educational, and belief systems differences.

As a starting point they present the three major domains of spirituality that promote connection (see Figure 1):

- *Beliefs* can be considered the cognitive dimension of spirituality, an affirmation of something considered real, which varies according to the individual's culture.

- *Practices* correspond to the dimension of behavior, being social or individual, public or private, requiring the engagement of the individual to perform activities such as meditating, praying, or going to meetings of a group that shares their spiritual or religious beliefs.

- *Experiences* compose the subjective aspect, based on the individual's perception of the presence of elements of interaction with the connecting object of spirituality, going beyond the bond of the intellect.

In the second axis (middle dark-gray section) are the possible aspects that can be connected through spiritual beliefs, practices, or experiences. These are classified as:

- *Sacred*, something that cannot be described in ordinary, profane terms. Something can be considered sacred through a manifestation, a revelation to the individual or their religious or spiritual group, such as an object or symbol that reveals something of a unique nature to the person who contemplates it.

- *Life after death*, related to the incorporeal, immaterial, and immortal portions present in the individual that survive in another realm after the body's

---

10 de Brito Sena, M. A., Damiano, R. F., Lucchetti, G., and Prieto Peres, M. F. (2021) "Defining spirituality in healthcare: A systematic review and conceptual framework." *Frontiers in Psychology 12*. https://doi.org/10.3389/fpsyg.2021.756080

death. This belief in the immortality of the soul, in the existence of a spiritual dimension, considering an extra-physical place, is found in some religions such as Catholicism, Judaism, Hinduism, and Buddhism.

- *Spiritual beings*, related to the contact or influence of immaterial beings, even ancestors, which can connect to the material world through a paranormal sensitivity or experiences of spirits or a supernatural presence.

- *Divine, God*, referring to the belief of one or more gods, beings of ultimate power connected to the celestial world, as a spirituality vertical dimension, and associated with a religious context.

- *Self*, relating to the connection with oneself, the body, and the individual's inner resources, or inner divinity.

- *Community*, aspects related to the ability to feel significant connection with other people in the community, neighbors, or family. This kind of connection could be understood as the social factor of spirituality.

- *Nature*, understanding the immanent nature as a means of expression of the sacred. It is already present in some Aboriginal cultures, Celtic, and folk religions, which respect all elements of nature as living beings.

- *Art*, contemplating or developing an artwork (painting, sculpture, music, dance, literature, architecture, etc.) is an aesthetic experience that can stimulate the individual's sensitive aspect, leading them to a state of awe and/or to the perception of transcendence. Art can be seen in some spiritual cultures and religious rituals, for example Buddhist sand mandalas and songs such as mantras.

The third axis (lower gray section) refers to the development of values, personal growth, and sensations of meaning, purpose in life, well-being, support, and inner peace through connection with something that can affect the behavior of the individual.

The identification of all these dimensions can be used by yoga therapists as an excellent tool in recognizing how their clients understand and express their spirituality.

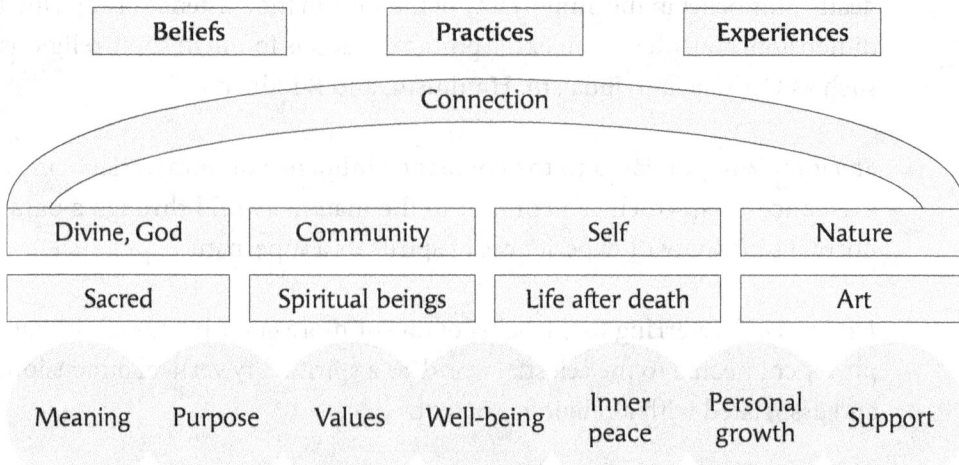

Figure 1. Spirituality framework proposition
*Source: de Brito Sena, M. A., Damiano, R. F., Lucchetti, G., and Prieto Peres, M. F. (2021)
"Defining spirituality in Healthcare: A systematic review and conceptual framework."
Frontiers in Psychology 12. https://doi.org/10.3389/fpsyg.2021.756080*

This growing interest in the subject of spirituality led, in 2011, to publication of the *Journal for the Study of Spirituality*, with two issues annually.[11] Their latest seminal publication, *The Routledge International Handbook of Spirituality in Society and the Professions*,[12] is over 450 pages long, containing articles from 68 contributing authors from all continents, making this a truly international endeavor, and proving that spirituality knows no boundaries—although this very thought gives rise to an interesting problem: How to define that which is boundless.

I am sure this is not the end of the evolution of our understanding of what spirituality is.

ASPECTS OF SPIRITUALITY

This interest in spirituality within the scientific and healthcare communities in the last two decades has led to a deeper comprehension of the subject, and brought about recognition of different aspects of spirituality, such as:

- *Spiritual care:* Defined as activities and methods to help patients face their fear of death, mitigate the uncertainty and discomfort of the treatment

---

11 www.tandfonline.com/loi/yjss20
12 Zsolnai, L. and Flanagan, B. (Eds) (2019) *The Routledge International Handbook of Spirituality in Society and the Professions*. London and New York: Routledge.

process, and regain their inner peace.[13] University Health Network (UHN) in Toronto, Canada, defines spiritual care "as care of individuals focusing on personal beliefs, core values, significant relationships, meanings, and behaviors around which we understand our lived experience,"[14] with spiritual care often delivered in healthcare systems by chaplains.

- *Spiritual health or well-being:* The state of an individual's understanding of the meaning of their own life; the value of themself, others, and the environment.[15] It can also be defined as expanding a sense of purpose and meaning in life, including an individual's morals and ethics. It may or may not involve religious activities.[16] In general terms, it is anything that relates to the health and wellness of a person's spirit. While spirit can be defined in many ways throughout many religions and cultures, the concept stems from something within an individual that cannot be seen in the body.

  Spiritual health or well-being is a facet of the self that connects to something larger than the person. It is just as important as mental and physical health because it is the way in which a person understands their place in the world, their purpose, and their reason for existing. Spiritual well-being can help people cope with stress, maintain psychological well-being, and in turn create healthy physical effects. It involves an individual being self-aware and knowing their meaning and purpose in life. It means people developing a better understanding of themselves, their personal beliefs, and what they value. In simple terms, it is about feeling grounded and connected—both in themselves and in the world.

- *Spiritual needs:* Expressed by lack of peace and hope, anger, of meaning of life, of fears, and loneliness. These can include:
  - To give and receive love
  - To be understood
  - To be valued as a human being

---

13 Appleby, A., Wilson, P., and Swinton, J. (2018) "Spiritual care in general practice: Rushing in or fearing to tread? An integrative review of qualitative literature." *Journal of Religion & Health 57*, 1108–1124. https://link.springer.com/article/10.1007/s10943-018-0583-5

14 UHN (University Health Network) (2022) *Spiritual Care: Spiritual and Religious Care for Patients, Families and Staff of UHN* [Brochure]. www.uhn.ca/PatientsFamilies/Health_Information/Health_Topics/Documents/Spiritual_Care.pdf

15 Li, X. H., Zhang, X. Q., Pan, Y. Q., *et al.* (2019) "Effect of cognitive adaptation process on spiritual well-being of patients with advanced lung cancer." *Guangdong Medical Journal*.

16 www.northwestern.edu/wellness

- Lack of forgiveness and trust
- To explore beliefs and values
- To find meaning, purpose, and hope.

• *Spiritual distress or crisis:* Defined as a state of inner suffering related to an inability to experience meaning in life, connection to self and/or others, the world and nature, and the superior being.[17] Spiritual distress can be experienced differently by different people. The use of indicators in diagnosing alterations in spiritual health is controversial because they may appear related to both spiritual and psychosocial problems.

  Signs and symptoms of spiritual distress may include:
  - Feelings of anger or hopelessness
  - Feelings of depression and anxiety
  - Difficulty sleeping
  - Feeling abandoned by God
  - Questioning the meaning of life or suffering
  - Questioning beliefs or sudden doubt in spiritual or religious beliefs
  - Asking why this situation occurred
  - Seeking spiritual help or guidance.

• *Spiritual pain:* A pain deep in the soul (being) that is non-physical, defined as a "self-identified experience of personal discomfort, or actual or potential harm, triggered by a threat to a person's relationship with God or a higher power."[18]

  Spiritual pain is often broken down into four categories:
  - Meaning—struggling with the "meaning" behind life, relationships, and the world around us
  - Forgiveness—pain that stems from forgiving others, ourselves, and God
  - Relatedness—dealing with relationships, whether good or bad
  - Hope—feeling like there is no hope, or that it doesn't exist at all.

• *Spiritual transformation or individuation:* Spiritual struggles often play a vital role in our spiritual development. They have been associated with

---

17 Eshghi, F., Nikfarid, L., and Zareiyan, A. (2023) "An integrative review of defining characteristic of the nursing diagnosis 'spiritual distress'." *Nursing Open 10*, 5, 2831–2841. https://pmc.ncbi.nlm.nih.gov/articles/PMC10077347

18 Illueca, M., Bradshaw, Y. S., and Carr, D. B. (2023) "Spiritual pain: A symptom in search of a clinical definition." *Journal of Religion and Health 62*, 3, 1920–1932. doi: 10.1007/s10943-022-01645-y.

increased symptoms of post-traumatic stress disorder (PTSD) and depression, and have been found to be followed by either a path of spiritual decline and hopelessness or a path of spiritual transformation and renewal.[19] Eckhart Tolle suggests that the destiny of human life is to awaken (develop or expand the consciousness), and the suffering is the spiritual teacher.

The path of renewal can lead to expansion of the consciousness, and may move an individual from one level of consciousness to another. Remember in Chapter 1 that we discussed Jim Marion's nine levels of consciousness, with level 4—the rational consciousness of teenagers and adults—being predominant in the masses. Level 5—vision-logic consciousness—Marion ascribes to the cutting edge of consciousness in the West today. This level invites us, as yoga therapists and practitioners, presumed consciousness pioneers, to enter. After all we have all the tools, as we will see in later chapters, to consciously work, through daily *sadhana (spiritual practice)*, on expanding our awareness by clearing our *kleshas* (the five human characteristics that cause human suffering, according to Patanjali's *Yoga Sutras*).

- *Spiritual intelligence:* This is the adaptive application of spirituality in life, which means the ability to use spirituality in everyday problem solving. It involves the ability to critically contemplate the nature of existence, the capacity to construct a life purpose and give meaning to daily chores and interactions, the ability to recognize transcendent dimensions of self or others, and of the environment, and finally, conscious state expansions—control over entering and exiting higher states of consciousness.[20]

    Spiritual intelligence is a skill, and like any other skill it can be developed through training by addressing and debating subjects such as self-awareness, self-management, self-consciousness, meaning in life, sense of holiness, and interpersonal relationships, as well as relaxation and meditation techniques. The benefits of such training are beyond doubt for the pregraduate curricula for any healthcare profession.[21] One study revealed that spiritual intelligence is a significant positive predictor of psychological well-being.

---

19 Barton, Y. A., Barkin, S. H., and Miller, L. (2017) "Deconstructing depression: A latent profile analysis of potential depressive subtypes in emerging adults." *Spirituality in Clinical Practice*. doi: 10.1037/scp0000126 fatcat:pi52ivxf55ez7hfiog4velsq6a.
20 King, D. B. (2008) "Rethinking Claims of Spiritual Intelligence: A Definition, Model and Measure" [Thesis]. Peterborough, Ontario, Canada.
21 Pinto, C. T., Veiga, F., Guedes, L. Ú., Pinto, S., and Nunes, R. (2023) "Models of spiritual intelligence interventions: A scoping review." *Nurse Education in Practice* 73, 103829. doi: 10.1016/j.nepr.2023.103829.

The results of this study provide "guidance" for educationalists who design activities for students entering the healthcare profession to increase their spiritual intelligence.[22]

- *Spiritual competence:* Spiritual intelligence is a cognitive foundation for spiritual competence development, enabling individuals to address their own beliefs and to be open to others. It is of major relevance for healthcare professionals, enabling them to answer a patient's spiritual needs in an empathic way.[23] Spiritual competence has been established as a core competency for palliative care professionals, and has seen its way into many nursing curricula worldwide.

I believe that both spiritual intelligence as well as spiritual competency training are a must for the curricula of any serious yoga therapy training. I would also add that any regulatory body of the yoga therapy profession should include these in the list of required competencies.

In her groundbreaking book *The Awakened Brain*,[24] published in mid-2021, Dr. Lisa Miller, an esteemed psychologist and award-winning researcher, presents a revolutionary exploration of the intersection between neuroscience and spirituality. This work represents a significant leap forward in our understanding of how spiritual experiences correlate with our biological processes. Dr. Miller's research, utilizing functional Magnetic Resonance Imaging (fMRI), focused on young people as they recounted spiritual experiences. The results were nothing short of remarkable, revealing a consistent connection between spiritual experiences and specific brain activity, regardless of the nature or context of these experiences.

The study identified two key brain networks associated with spiritual experiences:

- *Frontotemporal network:* When activated, participants reported physical sensations of warmth, calmness, increased energy, and a heightened sense of vitality.

---

22 Anwar, S. and Rana, H. (2023) "Spiritual intelligence and psychological wellbeing of Pakistani University students." *Current Psychology (New Brunswick, NJ)*, May 12, 1–8. doi: 10.1007/s12144-023-04717-8.

23 Hodge, D. R. (2016) "Spiritual competence: What it is, why it is necessary, and how to develop it." *Journal of Ethnic & Cultural Diversity in Social Work 27*, 2, 124–139. https://doi.org/10.1080/15313204.2016.1228093

24 Miller, L. (2021) *The Awakened Brain: The New Science of Spirituality and Our Quest for an Inspired Life.* New York: Random House.

- *Parietal lobe:* Activation in this area corresponded with emotional experiences such as clarity, awe, openness, peace, and a profound sense of connection with others, a higher power, or the environment.

Additionally, the ventral attention network—often referred to as the brain's "radar"—was engaged during moments of sudden guidance or insight. This network appears to be the source of those eureka moments and flashes of clarity that often accompany spiritual experiences.

Perhaps the most striking finding of Dr. Miller's research is the biological uniformity of intense spiritual awareness across the participants. Regardless of the specific nature of the experience, the brain activation patterns and levels of felt intensity were remarkably consistent. This suggests that we all possess a "spiritual part" of the brain that can be engaged intentionally, aligning with earlier work by Kendler and colleagues on the role of "deliberate inner life" in spiritual awakening.

Dr. Miller proposes that we have access to two distinct modes of awareness:

- *Achieving awareness:* This mode is task-oriented, focused on organizing and controlling our lives. It is characterized by a "doing" mindset and is crucial for goal attainment. However, when overused, it can lead to negative mental health outcomes. Here our foundational concern is, how can I get and keep what I want? This mode gives us focused attention and the commitment necessary to attain goals. It focuses our energy and attention on a particular task. We feel like makers of our path. We are in a "doing" mode.

- *Awakened awareness:* This mode utilizes different brain regions, allowing for a more integrated and holistic perception. It fosters creativity, connection, and a sense of life purpose. Literally we see more, integrating information from multiple sources of perception. This awareness allows us to perceive more choices and opportunities available to us, be more open to creative leaps and insights, and feel more in tune with our life's purpose and meaning. However, in this mode we do not lose or forsake our goals; we simply take off the blinders. Instead of seeing ourselves as independent makers of the path, we perceive ourselves as the seekers of our path. We are in a "being" mode.

Dr. Miller's research suggests that engaging our awakened awareness doesn't negate our goals but rather broadens our perspective. It allows us to reframe challenges within a larger context, potentially leading to more innovative solutions.

Importantly, Dr. Miller's study found that a "spiritual brain" is generally a healthier brain.

Dr. Miller offers practical ways to cultivate awakened awareness in daily life:

- *Awaken attention*—practice mindfulness and recognize synchronicities
- *Awaken heart*—foster altruism and compassion for others
- *Awaken connection*—cultivate a sense of oneness and transcendence.

These concepts align with theories of human consciousness evolution, suggesting that as we develop, we become less egocentric and more universally compassionate. The balance between achieving and awakened awareness may be a stepping stone to higher levels of consciousness, such as the psychic state described in Marion's scale of consciousness evolution.

In conclusion, Dr. Miller's work provides compelling evidence for the biological basis of spirituality, and offers a road map for integrating these insights into our daily lives, potentially paving the way for profound personal and societal transformation.

SPIRITUALITY AND HEALTH

Dr. Miller's work also implies that increased awareness influences the overall state of our health. To answer this question, let's turn our focus to healthcare, and specifically, the care provided to those nearing the end of life.

In the late 20th century, nurses and doctors working in palliative care were among the first to notice that patients with a strong sense of faith and community support found it easier to accept death.[25] These patients, regardless of their specific religious beliefs, often approached the end of life with peace and acceptance. Interestingly, even those who identified as atheists, but who had a sense of fulfillment or purpose in their lives, also faced death with a sense of calm.

However, patients without any religious or spiritual inclinations often experienced fear, anger, regret, and guilt as they confronted their mortality. It became evident that those who were spiritually inclined—whether religious or not—appeared to die with greater peace. Later research went on to confirm that spiritually inclined individuals not only faced death with more grace, but also healed faster from illnesses.[26]

---

25 Puchalski, C. M. (2015) "Spirituality in geriatric palliative care." *Clinics in Geriatric Medicine 31*, 2, 245–252. doi: 10.1016/j.cger.2015.01.011.

26 Torosian, M. H. and Biddle, V. R. (2005) "Spirituality and healing." *Seminars in Oncology 32*, 2, 232–236. https://doi.org/10.1053/j.seminoncol.2004.11.017

Despite these observations, the spiritual needs of patients were largely ignored by healthcare providers until the late 20th century. For much of history, spirituality was closely tied to religion, and the popular understanding of the term "spirituality" was often synonymous with religious practice. Even today, definitions such as those found in Merriam-Webster emphasize a connection to religious values or clergy. However, the *Encyclopedia Britannica* offers a more nuanced view, describing spirituality as not only related to religion but also as a capacity to grapple with fundamental questions about the nature of the self, the meaning of life, and consciousness. This expanded definition began to open the door to a more secular interpretation of spirituality.

Beginning around 1970, a few early research publications explored the relationship between health and spirituality, mostly from religious perspectives. By 1985, PubMed listed 174 articles discussing the influence of spirituality on health. By 1999, this number had grown to over 1400, with most studies published in medical and nursing journals rather than religious periodicals. The increasing emphasis on the role of spirituality in healthcare was a groundbreaking shift in understanding how deeply interconnected the mind, body, and spirit could be in the context of health.

A leading force in the movement to integrate spirituality into healthcare has been the GW Institute for Spirituality & Health (GWish).[27] Under the direction of Christina Puchalski, MD, GWish has played a pivotal role in "raising awareness of the importance of caring for the whole patient—physically, emotionally, socially, and spiritually." By conducting research, educating healthcare practitioners, and influencing healthcare policy, GWish has helped create more compassionate healthcare systems worldwide. The Institute frequently collaborates with religious, spiritual, and healthcare organizations to ensure that patients' spiritual needs are recognized and addressed.

One particularly notable study, published in 1997 by Kendler and colleagues,[28] was one of the first to explore whether there might be a genetic predisposition for spiritual experiences. The study involved over 1900 female twins, and sought to understand the relationship between religiosity, psychiatric symptoms, and the potential buffering effects of religious belief. It examined various factors, including religious beliefs, behaviors, and the conservatism of religious affiliations.

The results of the research were fascinating. Kendler and colleagues suggested

---

27 https://gwish.smhs.gwu.edu
28 Kendler, K. S., Gardner, C. O., and Prescott, C. A. (1997) "Religion, psychopathology, and substance use and abuse: A multimeasure, genetic-epidemiologic study." *American Journal of Psychiatry 154*, 322–329. https://doi.org/10.1176/ajp.154.3.322

that the capacity for a personal spiritual life was influenced by both heredity (29 percent) and environmental factors (71 percent). This finding highlighted the significant role that family, social environment, and cultural context play in shaping a person's spiritual life. More importantly, the study revealed that spirituality and religion are not the same: people could be spiritual without being religious, and vice versa. Furthermore, the study found that higher levels of spirituality were associated with lower risks of depression and addiction, offering a potential explanation for the success of 12-step programs, which are spiritual in nature. (We will explore these more closely in Chapter 3.)

In the past decades, several organizations (e.g., American College of Physicians, American Medical Association, American Nurses Association) have recognized the role of spirituality in clinical practice.[29] Likewise, this topic has been consistently incorporated into the curricula of several medical schools throughout the world, ranging from 40 percent of schools in Brazil to 59 percent of those in the UK, and 90 percent in the US.[30] This incorporation of spirituality into medical education has been prompted by the great number of publications and growing evidence of a relationship with health that has resulted in thousands of articles published in indexed scientific journals.

The relationship between spirituality and health has been also explored in a recent review published by Daniel *et al.* (2024).[31] Recognizing the role of spirituality in shaping health outcomes, they studied the existing research literature on the relationship between spirituality and three health outcomes:

- *Physical health outcomes*, such as mortality, morbidity, disease incidence, physiological functioning, and overall physical well-being. This includes longevity, the presence or absence of chronic diseases, disability, pain levels, and functional abilities.

- *Mental health outcomes*, such as emotional states, psychological well-being, and cognitive functioning. This includes levels of depression, anxiety, stress, resilience, and subjective well-being.

---

29 Moreira-Almeida, A., Koenig, H. G., and Lucchetti, G. (2014) "Clinical implications of spirituality to mental health: Review of evidence and practical guidelines." *Brazilian Journal of Psychiatry 36*, 2, 176–182. doi: 10.1590/1516-4446-2013-1255.

30 Neely, D. and Minford, E. J. (2008) "Current status of teaching on spirituality in UK medical schools." Medical Education 42, 2, 176–182. https://doi.org/10.1111/j.1365-2923.2007.02980.x

31 Alih, F., Daniel, S., and Halima, A. (2024) "The relationship between spirituality and health outcome." www.researchgate.net/publication/378942071

- *Social health outcomes*, which encompass an individual's social connections, relationships, and overall social functioning. This includes social support, social participation, community engagement, and the quality of interpersonal relationships.

Here are some of their key findings:

- *Physical health:* Some studies suggest a positive association between spirituality and physical health outcomes. For instance, some research has found that individuals who report higher levels of spirituality or religious involvement have lower rates of mortality, cardiovascular disease, and hypertension.[32] Spirituality has also been linked to better immune system functioning and improved pain management.[33]

- *Mental health:* Numerous studies have found that spirituality is associated with better mental health outcomes. For example, research has shown that individuals who engage in religious or spiritual practices have lower rates of depression, anxiety, and suicidal ideation.[34] They also tend to experience higher levels of life satisfaction, happiness, and overall psychological well-being.[35]

- *Coping with illness:* There is evidence to suggest that spirituality can play a significant role in coping with illness. Studies have shown that spirituality is associated with better psychological adjustment, improved quality of life, and enhanced resilience in the face of illness or chronic conditions. It can also influence treatment adherence and engagement in health-promoting behaviors.

- *Longevity:* Several studies have explored the relationship between spirituality

---

32 Balboni, T. A., VanderWeele, T. J., Doan-Soares, S. D., Long, K. N. G., et al. (2022) "Spirituality in serious illness and health." *JAMA 328*, 2, 184–197. doi: 10.1001/jama.2022.11086.
33 VanderWeele, T. J., Balboni, T. A., and Koh, H. K. (2017) "Health and spirituality." *JAMA 318*, 6, 519–520. doi: 10.1001/jama.2017.8136.
34 Milner, K., Crawford, P., Edgley, A., Hare-Duke, L., and Slade, M. (2019) "The experiences of spirituality among adults with mental health difficulties: A qualitative systematic review." *Epidemiology and Psychiatric Sciences 29*, e34. doi: 10.1017/S2045796019000234.
35 Sawab, S., Yusuf, A., Fitryasari, R., and Arifin, H. (2024) "Spirituality and recovery from severe mental disorders: A systematic review." *Journal of Psychosocial Nursing and Mental Health Services 62*, 8, 11–17. https://doi.org/10.3928/02793695-20240227-01

and longevity.[36] While the findings are mixed, some research suggests that individuals who engage in religious or spiritual practices tend to live longer. This association may be attributed to factors such as social support, healthier lifestyle choices, and enhanced coping mechanisms.

- *End-of-life care:* Spirituality has been found to have a positive impact on end-of-life care and the experience of dying. Studies have shown that spiritual beliefs and practices can help individuals find meaning, cope with the dying process, and experience a greater sense of peace and acceptance. Spiritual care interventions have also been shown to improve overall well-being and reduce psychological distress in palliative care settings.[37]

Another review studied the connection between spirituality and specific conditions.[38] Evidence has accumulated in recent years on the impact of spirituality and religiosity on various health outcomes related to longevity, including associations with decreased risk of mortality, cardiovascular disease, cancer, and cognitive decline, and healthy aging that leads to healthy longevity.

Some studies indicate that psychological well-being domains closely linked to spirituality may contribute to shape physical health. For example, two meta-analyses have shown that purpose in life and life satisfaction were associated with reduced mortality risk.[39] Contrariwise, social isolation and loneliness were related with increased mortality risk. Spirituality can be a source of comfort, hope, and inner peace, fostering a positive outlook on life that may lead to improved emotional and psychological well-being. Maintaining good mental health and a positive mindset has been linked to improved overall health and may indirectly influence longevity. In fact, spirituality, by enabling coping and overcoming negative events with meaning and purpose, has been associated with better mental health (lower rates of depression, less anxiety, less stress, greater well-being, and positive emotions).

---

36 Buja, A., Grotto, G., and Vo, D. (2024) "Association of religiosity and spirituality with survival among older adults: A systematic review." *Journal of Public Health (Berlin).* https://doi.org/10.1007/s10389-024-02303-1

37 Soffer, E. D. (2024) "The lived spiritual experience of aging adults (≥65)." Dissertation, Walden University. https://scholarworks.waldenu.edu/cgi/viewcontent.cgi?article=17013&context=dissertations

38 Dominguez, L. J., Veronese, N., and Barbagallo, M. (2023) "The link between spirituality and longevity." *Aging Clinical and Experimental Research 36*, 32. https://doi.org/10.1007/s40520-023-02684-5

39 Collet, R., van Grootel, J., van Dongen, J., Wiertsema, S., *et al.* (2025) "The impact of multidisciplinary transitional care interventions for complex care needs: A systematic review and meta-analysis." *Gerontologist* March 5, gnaf088. doi: 10.1093/geront/gnaf088; Boehm, J. K., Winning, A., Segerstrom, S., and Kubzansky, L. D. (2015) "Variability modifies life satisfaction's association with mortality risk in older adults." *Psychological Science 26*, 7, 1063–1070. doi: 10.1177/0956797615581491.

By promoting overall mental well-being, spiritual practices may directly influence several biological systems, including the sympathetic nervous, endocrine, and immune systems. Acute and chronic dysregulation of the stress system at different levels has been implicated as a major pathway and link to numerous behavioral (e.g., anxiety, depression, eating disorders, PTSD, sleep disorders, etc.) and somatic disorders (e.g., chronic pain and fatigue syndromes, obesity, metabolic syndrome, chronic inflammation, type 2 diabetes, hypertension (HTN), atherosclerosis, and cardiovascular diseases). Some studies also show the positive effects of meditation on objective measurements such as a reduction of blood cortisol levels in the short and long term, as reported in a recent meta-analysis.[40]

A recent cross-sectional study evaluated HTN for four racial/ethnic groups and diverse spirituality variables[41], including individual prayer, group prayer, nontheistic daily spiritual experiences, yoga, gratitude, and positive and negative religious coping. This study found different patterns of associations depending on gender and ethnicity. Among women: (1) religious attendance was associated with lower HTN among Black and white women; (2) gratitude was linked to lower HTN among Hispanic/Latino, South Asian, and white women; (3) individual prayer was associated with higher HTN prevalence among Hispanic/Latino and white women; (4) yoga was associated with higher HTN among South Asian women; and (5) negative religious coping was linked to higher HTN among Black women.

Some studies have evaluated the association of spirituality and the incidence of cancer or outcomes in patients with cancer[42]; 55 percent found that those with more spiritual practices had a lower risk of developing cancer, or a better prognosis when already diagnosed with it.

With an increasingly aging population, interest has grown globally in identifying factors that may contribute to healthy aging and healthy longevity. Key aspects of the role that spirituality may play in promoting healthy aging include increased social support, the associations with improved quality of life, decreased mortality, and reduction of some chronic conditions, psychological and mental health and resilience, purpose in life, improved cognitive function, and better management of end-of-life and issues around death.

---

40 Koncz, A., Demetrovics, Z., and Takacs, Z. K. (2020) "Meditation interventions efficiently reduce cortisol levels of at-risk samples: A meta-analysis." *Health Psychology Review 15*, 1, 56–84. doi: 10.1080/17437199.2020.1760727

41 Kent, B. K., Upenieks, L., Kanaya, A. M., Warner, E. T., *et al.* (2023) "Religion/spirituality and prevalent hypertension among ethnic cohorts in the study on stress, spirituality and health." *Annals of Behavioral Medicine 57*, 8, 649–661. doi: 10.1093/abm/kaad007

42 Dominguez, L. J., Veronese, N., and Barbagallo, M. (2023) "The link between spirituality and longevity." *Aging Clinical and Experimental Research 36*, 32. https://doi.org/10.1007/s40520-023-02684-5

Analyses from the Nurses' Health Study[43] reported that women who were more socially integrated were more likely to be healthy agers (no history of major chronic disease diagnosis, no self-reported impairment in memory, and no major impairments in physical function or mental health). However, while there might be some correlations between spirituality and health outcomes, they do not necessarily imply causation, and not all spiritual beliefs or practices are beneficial for everyone: there is no "one-size-fits-all" approach to spirituality.

It is essential to remember that there are significant differences in terms of sex, ethnicity, cultural background, education, and characteristics of family nuclei and communities regarding the interpretation of the role that spirituality can play in healthy aging. This may generate profound difficulties in applying spiritual interventions that can help in promoting healthy longevity.

A very interesting review of the assessment of spirituality in mental health presented an historical perspective of a psychiatric understanding of spirituality.[44] It mentions that in the 19th and 20th centuries, particularly in the field of psychiatry, spiritual and religious involvement was viewed as negative and responsible for worse outcomes, such as hysteria and neurosis. This created a separation between spirituality/religion and medicine, and has resulted in negative attitudes toward addressing spiritual and religious beliefs in clinical practice.

In the 1970s and 1980s, however, several studies were published showing that spirituality and religiosity were generally associated with better mental health.[45] Following these, psychiatry residency programs began incorporating this topic into their curricula. Yet it took another 30 years before the World Psychiatry Association published (in 2016) a position statement on spirituality and religion urging the inclusion of both on clinical encounters and training, with the goal of providing a more holistic and comprehensive form of mental healthcare.[46]

Here is a summary of the results as correlated to spirituality and specific mental issues:

---

43 Li, S., Hagan, K., Grodstein, F., and VanderWeele, T. J. (2018) "Social integration and healthy aging among US women." *Preventive Medicine Reports 9*, 144–148. doi: 10.1016/j.pmedr.2018.01.013

44 Hirshbein, L. (2020) "Religion and Spirituality, Meaning, and Faith in American Psychiatry From the 19th to the 21st Century." *J Nerv Ment Dis., 208*, 8, 582–586. doi: 10.1097/NMD.0000000000001191

45 See, for example, McCullough, M. E., Hoyt, W. T., Larson, D. B., Koenig, H. G., and Thoresen, C. (2000) "Religious involvement and mortality: A meta-analytic review." *Health Psychology 19*, 3, 211–222. doi: 10.1037//0278-6133.19.3.211.

46 Moreira-Almeida, A., Sharma, A., van Rensburg, B. J., Verhagen, P. J., and Cook, C. C. H. (2016) "WPA Position Statement on spirituality and religion in psychiatry." *World Psychiatry 15*, 1, 87–88. doi: 10.1002/wps.20304.

- *Depression:* A higher level of spirituality is generally associated with lower depressive symptoms in Western countries. However, a 13-year-long study, which investigated over 67,000 adults in Japan, found that highly religious individuals had more major depressive disorders compared to nonreligious individuals.[47] Such discrepancy in outcomes has been confirmed in other studies. This indicates that cultural, ethnographic, and educational difference may explain differences in outcomes.

- *Suicide:* A higher level of spirituality is generally associated with lower rates of suicide attempts and completed suicide.[48] Large studies specifically point to religious attendance, but not religious affiliation, as protective against suicide in Western countries.[49]

- *Substance use disorder:* There is robust evidence that a higher level of spirituality/religiosity is generally associated with lower substance use.[50] Although studies on spirituality/religiosity and alcohol use or abuse are more common, the same findings are also being reported for other substances.[51]

- *Psychotic disorder:* Patients with psychotic disorders can present with religious delusions that are sometimes difficult to distinguish from nonpsychotic religious beliefs. Evidence shows that religious delusions have been associated with poor functioning, longer duration of illness, and more severe symptoms.[52] Often, but not always, these occur in highly religious

---

47 Kobayashi, D., First, M. B., Shimbo, T., Kanba, S., and Hirano, Y. (2020) "Association of self-reported religiosity with the development of major depression in multireligious country Japan." *Psychiatry and Clinical Neurosciences 74*, 10, 535–541. doi: 10.1111/pcn.13087.

48 Lucchetti, G., Koenig, H. G., and Lucchetti, A. L. G. (2021) "Spirituality, religiousness, and mental health: A review of the current scientific evidence." *World Journal of Clinical Cases 9*, 26, 7620–7631. doi: 10.12998/wjcc.v9.i26.7620

49 O'Reilly, D. and Rosato, M. (2015) "Religion and the risk of suicide: Longitudinal study of over 1 million people." *The British Journal of Psychiatry 206*, 6, 466–470. https://doi.org/10.1192/bjp.bp.113.128694

50 Lucchetti, G., Koenig, H. G., and Lucchetti, A. L. G. (2021) "Spirituality, religiousness, and mental health: A review of the current scientific evidence." *World Journal of Clinical Cases 9*, 26, 7620–7631. doi: 10.12998/wjcc.v9.i26.7620

51 Orme-Johnson, D. W. (1994). "Transcendental Meditation as an epidemiological approach to drug and alcohol abuse: theory, research, and financial impact evaluation." *Alcoholism Treatment Quarterly*, 11, 119–168.

52 Iyassu, R., Jolley, S., Bebbington, P., Dunn, G., et al. (2013) "Psychological characteristics of religious delusions." *Social Psychiatry and Psychiatric Epidemiology 49*, 7, 1051–1061. doi: 10.1007/s00127-013-0811-y

patients. Nonpsychotic religious beliefs and spirituality are generally associated with better social, clinical, and psychological outcomes.

- *Obsessive compulsive disorder (OCD):* Only a few studies are available that indicate both positive and negative outcomes.

- *Bipolar disorder:* Although only a few studies are available, a higher level of spirituality is generally associated with better outcomes.

- *PTSD:* Studies involving survivors of the Covid-19 pandemic,[53] the war in Bosnia-Herzegovina,[54] and adolescents in the Gaza strip[55] strongly indicate that spirituality may serve to buffer against PTSD, generally increasing psychological growth following a stressful situation.

- *Eating disorders:* The relationship between spirituality/religiosity and eating disorders is probably one of the most unexplored areas in spirituality/religiosity and mental health. Most of the studies involve small convenience samples or case reports. However, a recent systematic review on this topic summarizes the results from 22 studies, finding strong positive religious/spiritual beliefs associated with lower levels of disordered eating and body image concerns.[56]

There is no single mechanism to explain the effects of spirituality on mental health. Koenig[57] proposed that spirituality is associated with human virtues (e.g., forgiveness, altruism, gratefulness), and that these virtues may mediate the relationship between spirituality and mental health outcomes. Attempts have recently been

---

53 Xiao, W., Liu, X., Wang, H., Huang, Y., *et al.* (2023) "Prevalence and risk for symptoms of PTSD among survivors of a COVID-19 infection." *Psychiatry Research 326*, 115304. doi: 10.1016/j.psychres.2023.115304.

54 Comtesse, H., Powell, S., Soldo, A., Hagl, M., and Rosner, R. (2019) "Long-term psychological distress of Bosnian war survivors: An 11-year follow-up of former displaced persons, returnees, and stayers." *BMC Psychiatry 19*, 1, 1. doi: 10.1186/s12888-018-1996-0.

55 El-Khodary, B., Samara, M., and Askew, C. (2020) "Traumatic events and PTSD among Palestinian children and adolescents: The effect of demographic and socioeconomic factors." *Frontiers in Psychiatry 11*, 4. doi: 10.3389/fpsyt.2020.00004.

56 Akrawi, D., Bartrop, R., Potter, U., and Touyz, S. (2015) "Religiosity, spirituality in relation to disordered eating and body image concerns: A systematic review." *Journal of Eating Disorders 3*, 29. doi: 10.1186/s40337-015-0064-0.

57 Koenig, H. G. (2012) "Religion, spirituality, and health: The research and clinical implications." *ISRN Psychiatry* 278730. doi: 10.5402/2012/278730.

made to identify specific markers that may help to explain the relationship between spirituality and mental health. Higher levels of spirituality have been associated with higher rates of brain-derived neurotrophic factor;[58] self-transcendence has been linked to serotonin transporter (SERT) availability in brainstem raphe nuclei;[59] and correlations have been reported between spirituality and genes for dopamine, serotonin, vesicular transporters, and oxytocin.[60]

In fact, research shows that engaging in spiritual practices—whether through organized religion or more individualized approaches—has profound implications for both physical and mental health.[61] Studies have found that people who regularly engage in spiritual practices tend to live longer and report higher levels of life satisfaction and purpose.[62] This suggests that spirituality is not just an abstract concept, but a vital component of overall well-being.

These findings have important clinical implications. Previous studies have shown that patients have spiritual needs that they wish to be addressed by health professionals. Few health professionals, however, bring up spirituality issues during clinical encounters,[63] and the situation is even worse among psychiatrists. Based on this review of the research, spirituality has an important influence, one way or another, on mental health outcomes. In the next chapter we will examine more closely how our spiritual needs are met in the healthcare environment, as well as present examples of how secular spirituality is still present in our lives.

---

58   Mosqueiro, B. P., Fleck, M. P., and da Rocha, N. S. (2019) "Increased levels of brain-derived neurotrophic factor are associated with high intrinsic religiosity among depressed inpatients." *Frontiers in Psychiatry 10*, 671. doi: 10.3389/fpsyt.2019.00671.

59   Kim, J. H., Son, Y. D., Kim, J. H., Choi, E. J., *et al.* (2015) "Self-transcendence trait and its relationship with *in vivo* serotonin transporter availability in brainstem raphe nuclei: An ultra-high resolution PET-MRI study." *Brain Research 1629*, 63–71. https://doi.org/10.1016/j.brainres.2015.10.006

60   Anderson, M. R., Miller, L., Wickramaratne, P., Svob, C., *et al.* (2017) "Genetic correlates of spirituality/religion and depression: A study in offspring and grandchildren at high and low familial risk for depression." *Spirituality in Clinical Practice (Washington DC) 4*, 1, 43–63. doi: 10.1037/scp0000125.

61   Malviya, S. (2023) "The need for integration of religion and spirituality into the mental health care of culturally and linguistically diverse populations in Australia: A rapid review." *Journal of Religion and Health 62*, 4, 2272–2296. doi: 10.1007/s10943-023-01761-3.

62   Alih, F., Daniel, S., and Halima, A. (2024) "The relationship between spirituality and health outcome." www.researchgate.net/publication/378942071

63   Best, M., Butow, P., and Olver, I. (2016) "Doctors discussing religion and spirituality: A systematic literature review." *Palliative Medicine 30*, 4, 327–337. doi: 10.1177/0269216315600912.

CHAPTER 3

Is Secular Spirituality Alive?

The most beautiful thing we can experience is the mysterious. It is the source of all true art and science.

ALBERT EINSTEIN (1879–1955)

In Chapter 2 we explored how spirituality has evolved over time and how it has been understood in various contexts. Yet despite this evolution, many people today still struggle to articulate what spirituality means outside the framework of organized religion. This confusion is understandable, as spirituality is deeply personal and often difficult to express in simple terms. However, it is important to recognize that spirituality has always been an intrinsic part of human life, whether we are consciously aware of it or not. It lives in our myths, folk tales, and cultural traditions, even if it isn't explicitly labeled as "spiritual."

Yet these days, and particularly in high-income countries, such as those in Europe and North America, religiosity is on the decline. A growing number of people identify as atheists or agnostics, leaving traditional religious institutions unable to fill the spiritual void as they once did. But this does not mean that spirituality has disappeared from people's lives—perhaps it has simply taken on new forms. As we will see in this chapter, people look for these experiences in everyday activities, often without realizing why they like them.

Let us remind ourselves that, according to Dr. Miller, spiritual experience is visible in the brain in three ways:

- An involuntary reorientation of attention
- A sense of love consistent with intimate bonding
- A sense of self that is both distinct and part of the greater oneness (self-transcending awareness).

Spiritual experience physically produced the feelings of warmth, calmness, heightened energy, and aliveness. Participants in Dr. Miller's research experienced clarity, awe, openness, peace, and unity. Boundaries dissolved and a feeling of oneness with the divine or environment developed. *Spirituality is our innate capacity that protects our mental health.* We're hardwired to awaken, transform, and expand, even through trauma. Spiritual awakening therefore depends more on the deliberate use of our inner life.

As we will see, people continue to seek out these experiences in many ways. It may be through practices such as yoga, tai chi, and meditation, connecting with nature, or participating in community activities such as music-making or volunteer work. These activities may not always be recognized as "spiritual" in the conventional sense, but they serve similar functions—they give us experiences of being connected to ourselves, to others, and to something greater than ourselves. Many of us look for these deeper experiences often without realizing that they are fulfilling our spiritual needs.

SPIRITUALITY IN HEALTHCARE

The integration of spirituality into healthcare has gained significant attention in recent years. Studies have shown that regular participation in spiritual or religious practices can have tangible effects on health outcomes.[1,2] For example, attending religious services has been linked to lower rates of mortality from all causes, including cardiovascular diseases and cancer. This suggests that spirituality may serve as a protective factor against major health risks.

But why does this connection exist? One possible explanation is that spiritual practices often promote a sense of community, belonging, and purpose—factors that are known to enhance mental well-being. The social support inherent in religious or spiritual communities can buffer individuals against stress, which is a major contributor to many chronic illnesses. Additionally, spiritual practices often encourage mindfulness, meditation, or prayer—all of which have been shown to reduce stress hormones like cortisol and improve overall mental health.

However, healthcare providers often face challenges when trying to integrate spirituality into patient care. Time constraints and heavy workloads make it

---

1   Li, S., Stampfer, M. J., Williams, D. R., and VanderWeele, T. J. (2016) "Association of religious service attendance with mortality among women." *JAMA Internal Medicine* 176, 6, 777–785. doi: 10.1001/jamainternmed.2016.1615.
2   Cohen, R., Bavishi, C., and Rozanski, A. (2016) "Purpose in life and its relationship to all-cause mortality and cardiovascular events: A meta-analysis." *Psychosomatic Medicine* 78, 2, 122–133. doi: 10.1097/PSY.0000000000000274.

difficult for doctors and nurses to engage in meaningful conversations about a patient's spiritual needs. Moreover, many healthcare professionals receive limited training in cultural competence or integrating spirituality into medical care. This gap highlights the importance of chaplaincy services in hospitals, where trained professionals can provide spiritual care tailored to each patient's needs.

Chaplaincy has evolved significantly over the years, and has become an important part of healthcare, providing a spiritual service to patients and their families. Initially rooted in Christian traditions, modern chaplaincy now embraces a more inclusive approach that addresses the spiritual needs of people from diverse backgrounds and belief systems.[3] Chaplains are trained not only to offer prayers or religious rites, but also to listen empathetically and help patients navigate existential questions about life, death, and suffering. This shift towards a more holistic model of chaplaincy reflects broader changes in society's understanding of spirituality. As fewer people identify with organized religion—especially in high-income countries—there is a growing need for spiritual care that transcends traditional religious boundaries. Chaplains today are equipped to work with patients who may not identify with any particular faith, but who still seek meaning and comfort during times of illness or crisis.

In critical care situations or end-of-life settings, chaplains often serve as vital links between patients, families, and medical staff.[4] They help facilitate difficult conversations about treatment options or palliative care while providing emotional support to both patients and their loved ones. In doing so, chaplains play an essential role in ensuring that healthcare is not just about treating physical ailments but also addressing the emotional and spiritual dimensions of healing. It is worth noting, for example, that in 2008 chaplaincy services were provided at approximately only 68 percent of all hospitals in the US,[5] and these were mostly in large hospitals, with smaller hospitals relying on local pastoral and volunteer services.

You may think that spiritual needs only come to play in a crisis, such as a serious disease needing hospitalization or end-of-life settings in a hospice. Let us now consider if there are other everyday situations where spirituality may play an important role in our lives.

---

3   Gleason, J. J. (1998) "An emerging paradigm in professional chaplaincy." *Chaplaincy Today* 14, 2, 9–14. https://doi.org/10.1080/10999183.1998.10767090
4   Gillman, J., Gable-Rodriguez, J., Sutherland, S. M., and Whitacre, R. J. (1996) "Pastoral care in a critical care setting." *Critical Care Nursing Quarterly* 19, 1, 10–20. doi: 10.1097/00002727-199605000-00004.
5   Cadge, W., Freese, J., and Christakis, N. A. (2008) "The provision of hospital chaplaincy in the United States: A national overview." *Southern Medical Journal* 101, 6, 626–630. doi: 10.1097/SMJ.0b013e3181706856.

SPIRITUALITY BEYOND CRISIS: EVERYDAY APPLICATIONS

Imagine standing at the edge of a vast wilderness, the wind rustling through ancient trees, and a sense of something greater than yourself washing over you. This isn't just poetic fancy; it's a very real experience for many who venture into nature's domain.

In 1999, researchers in Ontario, Canada, decided to put numbers to this feeling. They asked over 11,000 visitors to provincial parks about their spiritual experiences. Surprisingly, more than half of these everyday adventurers reported that spirituality significantly enhanced their park visit.[6] It seems that the great outdoors has a knack for nurturing our inner lives.

But what exactly happens when we step into nature's cathedral? Researchers suggest it's a bit like peeling an onion.[7] First, the stress of daily life falls away. As we relax, we become more open to deeper experiences. Suddenly, the rustling leaves might speak to our inner selves, or a majestic vista could stir profound emotions. These aren't just fleeting moments of awe. Over time, these experiences can lead to genuine spiritual growth. It's as if nature provides a gentle on-ramp to the transcendent.

A team from the University of Haifa in Israel wanted to understand this phenomenon better.[8] They spoke with wilderness guides from around the world, seasoned experts in facilitating these nature–spirit connections. Their findings paint a vivid picture of how we experience spirituality in the wild:

- *Nature as spiritual embodiment:* The physical world becomes a tangible link to the mysterious. You don't need to be religious to feel it—it's as natural as breathing in the forest air. The expansion of consciousness, the study suggests, is attained by deeply connecting with physical, wild, and sensual experiences.

- *Expanding perspectives:* Standing before a vast landscape can shift our viewpoint dramatically. Suddenly, our personal stories fit into a much larger

---

6   Heintzman, P. (2010) "Leisure studies and spirituality: A Christian critique." *Movement and Being: The Journal of the Christian Society for Kinesiology, Leisure and Sports Studies 1*, 1, Article 2. https://trace.tennessee.edu/cgi/viewcontent.cgi?article=1003&context=jcskls
7   Fox, R. (1999) "Enhancing spiritual experience in adventure programs." In J. C. Miles and S. Priest (Eds) *Adventure Programming* (pp.455–461). State College, PA: Venture.
8   Naor, L. and Mayseless, O. (2020) "The therapeutic value of experiencing spirituality in nature." *Spirituality in Clinical Practice 7*, 2, 114–133. https://doi.org/10.1037/scp0000204

narrative. The connection with that which is greater than us and is eternal and infinite appears to allow a new, more expansive perspective and perhaps meaning of life. This resonates with psychological notions that emphasize the importance of spirituality as nurturing the human desire to find meaning within the reality of our own mortality.

- *Deep belonging:* Nature reminds us that we are part of an intricate web of life. This realization can provide a profound sense of purpose and connection. This allows us to view everything in nature as sentient, relating and connecting with everything else. When we recognize and relate to this, we begin to accept ourselves as part of this interconnected world, and our participation and belonging gain meaning and purpose.

- *Nature as a mirror:* The wilderness often reflects our inner truths back to us, leading to moments of profound self-discovery. When we perceive ourselves as part of nature, we perceive specific occurrences and elements in nature as reflecting relevant personal information. The wilderness guides described this as a unique mirroring occurring in nature, evoking a unique discovery process, allowing them to know who they were.

These spiritual experiences in nature aren't just feel-good moments; they appear to have real therapeutic value. Australian researchers found that people who felt more connected to nature reported greater life satisfaction.[9] This spiritual connection seems to act as a bridge, linking experiences of nature to improved psychological well-being.

Perhaps most remarkably, a decade of research has failed to find any group that doesn't benefit from contact with nature.[10] In our increasingly urbanized world, this suggests that maintaining a connection to the natural world isn't just nice to have; it's essential for our health and happiness.

Spirituality in nature offers something unique. It exists in a space between traditional religious practices and the realm of scientific inquiry. For many, it provides a way to explore the deeper questions of existence without the constraints

---

9   Kamitis, I. and Francis, A. J. P. (2013) "Spirituality mediates the relationship between engagement with nature and psychological wellbeing." *Journal of Environmental Psychology* 36, 136–143. http://dx.doi.org/10.1016/j.jenvp.2013.07.013
10 Pretty, J., Rogerson, M., and Barton, J. (2017) "Green mind theory: How brain-body-behaviour links into natural and social environments for healthy habits." *International Journal of Environmental Research and Public Health* 14, 7, 706. doi: 10.3390/ijerph14070706.

of dogma or the cold logic of pure rationality. As we face growing environmental challenges, perhaps this spiritual connection to nature could play a crucial role. By fostering a deeper, more meaningful relationship with the natural world, we might find not only personal healing but also the motivation to protect the very landscapes that nourish our souls.

In the end, the wilderness isn't just calling us to adventure; it's inviting us to rediscover an essential part of our humanity. So the next time you feel the urge to take a walk in the woods or gaze at a starry sky, remember—you might just be answering a call as old as humanity itself—which I found very helpful in my personal life.

As a single parent working in the corporate world and under constant stress, I had only two weeks of time off alone a year. For years I would spend those two summer weeks in the backcountry, camping and canoeing, alone in total wilderness, where I had no contact with any humans. It usually took me three days to shed off the city and feel at one with the surrounding nature. Interestingly, over these three days, I could feel myself slowly switching from constant rushed activities, from "doing," to appreciative "beingness." After these three days, time seemed to collapse; there would be no thoughts of the past or future as I felt myself an integral yet insignificant part of the environment. Two weeks of such "therapy" would reset and restore me completely.

I used another "application" of spirituality in nature with my husband in times of conflict. We would agree to leave the matter until we could go for an extended walk in nature. After half an hour of being in a park, we would start discussing the point of contention. The initial 30 minutes of silently walking together in such an environment caused our voices to mellow; we would find it easy to suspend our judgments and to fully listen to the other side. It felt like we both moved to more expanded consciousness, which made us both see the bigger perspective and loosen our grip on our own opposing positions. It became much easier to find a mutually agreeable solution in situations where we initially thought there was no way out of the conflict.

SPIRITUALITY IN A COMMUNITY OF SHARED INTERESTS

It is interesting to consider how communities form, often not around spiritual subjects or activities but through shared experiences that foster deep interpersonal connections. These connections can grow so strong that they naturally lead the group toward a sense of spirituality, even if that wasn't the original intention. This kind of community can take many shapes, with members sharing different interests, but still finding a sense of unity and purpose.

One particularly fascinating example of this is a choir. A choir brings together synchronized individual participation, music as a spiritual medium, and a harmonized group effort. Research by Hills and Argyle offered an insightful comparison between musical and spiritual experiences.[11] They found that both can evoke powerful emotions—intense yet personal feelings that occur in public settings like worship services or choral concerts. Both music and spirituality can lift moods and create positive emotional states. In their study, Hills and Argyle surveyed 11 items related to musical experiences, and nine of these showed greater intensity in the context of music-making. Six were statistically significant, with the most common feelings being upliftment, joy, and the shared elation that comes from performing together.

If we think about spirituality as central to finding meaning and purpose in life, then music becomes a bridge to those goals. Participating in communal music activities—especially in a choir—can be a path to discovering our authentic self. This journey is also a key aspect of music therapy, where music acts as a vehicle for healing and self-discovery. The paradox here is that while music can create deeply personal spiritual experiences, it often does so most powerfully when shared with others.

Many types of musical groups offer benefits—string quartets, symphonies, concert bands—but there is something unique about being part of a choir. Silber captures this beautifully: while any group musical activity can help develop interpersonal skills, multipart singing demands something special.[12] It creates complex relational dynamics as singers must balance their individual voices with those around them—a perfect metaphor for relationships themselves. In a choir, each singer must control their own voice while blending harmoniously with others. This requires not only technical skill but also patience, self-control, intuition, and trust. It's about listening closely to others while contributing our own part to create something greater than the sum of its parts—a harmonic whole.

Historically, choirs have played many roles in society. From ritual chants in ancient religious ceremonies to Gregorian chants in early Christian worship, choirs have long been associated with spiritual communion. Over time, these simple chants evolved into more complex forms of music that fostered a sense of unity among participants.

---

11 Hills, P. and Argyle, M. (1998) "Musical and religious experiences and their relationship to happiness." *Personality and Individual Differences* 25, 1, 91–102. https://doi.org/10.1016/S0191-8869(98)00004-X

12 Silber, L. (2005) "Bars behind bars: The impact of a women's prison choir on social harmony." *Music Education Research* 7, 2, 251–271. https://doi.org/10.1080/14613800500169811

Choirs have also played important social roles outside religious contexts. For example, during the era of slavery in the American South, call-and-response singing on plantations helped create solidarity among workers. The songs were initiated by a soloist and echoed by the group—a powerful way to foster community through collective singing.

The choral movement has continued to grow globally since the Second World War. In 1960, the European Federation of Youth Choruses (EFYC) was founded in Geneva, connecting over 2.5 million people across more than 50 countries. Similar associations have since sprung up worldwide—America Cantat, Asia Cantat, Africa Cantat—all celebrating choral music as a symbol of solidarity and peace.

Today, choral singing is one of the most common forms of musical participation in many parts of the world, with particularly strong choral traditions in Northern Europe. In the US, choral singing is widespread across towns and cities.[13] In Canada there are about 50 percent more adult choral singers than hockey players, with one in every 15 adults singing in a choir.[14] About one in four Canadian children sing in a choir, three times more than play hockey. Considering the Canadian national craze with hockey, these statistics say a lot for choir attendance.

So why this global explosion of choirs? A 2012 study surveyed over 1100 choral singers from Australia, England, and Germany to explore the benefits of choral singing.[15] The results were remarkable, with participants reporting:

- Numerous social benefits (networking opportunities and a sense of belonging)
- Mood benefits (feeling energized and relaxed)
- Even physiological benefits (improved respiratory health and stress reduction).

Another study involving over 1700 participants from 19 countries confirmed these findings: singing was consistently seen as spiritually uplifting and life-affirming.[16] Choirs provided an outlet for creativity while fostering deep connections with others.

---

13 Chorus America: www.chorusamerica.org
14 https://hillstrategies.com/resource/choral-singing-choral-attendance-and-the-situation-of-choirs-in-canada
15 Livesey, L., Morrison, I., Clift, S., and Camic, P. (2012) "Benefits of choral singing for social and mental wellbeing: Qualitative findings from a cross-national survey of choir members." *Journal of Public Mental Health 11*, 1, 10–26. https://doi.org/10.1108/17465721211207275
16 Moss, H., Lynch, J., and O'Donoghue, J. M. (2018) "Exploring the perceived health benefits of singing in a choir: An international cross-sectional mixed-methods study." *Perspectives in Public Health 138*, 3. https://doi.org/DOI: 10.1177/1757913917739652

Interestingly enough, after Covid-19 lockdowns ended in Sweden and Norway, researchers asked over 5000 amateur singers what they missed most during isolation.[17] The overwhelming response? Social bonding through communal activity. Singing together stimulates oxytocin—the "cuddle hormone" associated with trust—and creates moments of "flow," where participants are fully absorbed in their activity without feeling mental effort.

Personally speaking—as someone who has sung in choirs for most of my life—I can attest to these profound experiences firsthand. There's something magical about being part of a choir: moments when you lose yourself entirely in the music and feel connected to something much larger than yourself. It's as if the choir becomes one body—an experience so deeply spiritual that words often fail to capture its essence.

SPIRITUALITY IN ADDICTION AND RECOVERY

One recovery program talks about a human need to fill the "hole in the soul." This phrase captures a deep, almost universal human urge to become all that we are capable of being. When this need goes unrecognized, it can lead to a profound sense of existential pain—a feeling that something essential is missing. Without understanding the source of this discomfort, people often turn to various activities to numb the pain. These can include work, substance use, drugs, alcohol, food, gambling, and more. Over time, these behaviors can become addictive, slowly eroding a person's health, and even threatening their life.

Addiction has been recognized as a public health crisis in Canada since 2016.[18] In the US, drug abuse and addiction remain overwhelming issues for the healthcare system. According to AddictionHelp.com, 25.4 percent of illicit drug users suffer from dependency or addiction. Of the nearly 140 million people aged 12 and older who drink alcohol, over 20 percent struggle with alcohol abuse or addiction. Additionally, about half of individuals diagnosed with a mental illness will also face substance abuse at some point in their lives—and vice versa.[19] Globally, Statista.com estimates that there are around 39.5 million individuals addicted to illegal drugs.[20]

---

17 Askim, J. and Bergström, T. (2021) "Between lockdown and calm down: Comparing the COVID-19 responses of Norway and Sweden." *Local Government Studies 48*, 2, 291–311. https://doi.org/10.1 080/03003930.2021.1964477
18 Snodgrass, S., Corcoran, L., and Jerry, P. (2024) "Spirituality in addiction recovery: A narrative review." *Journal of Religion and Health 63*, 1, 515–530. doi: 10.1007/s10943-023-01854-z.
19 USA addiction statistics: www.addictionhelp.com/addiction/statistics/#:~:text=13.5%25%20of%20 Americans%2012%20and,from%20alcohol%20abuse%20or%20addiction
20 Statista Research Department (2024) "Global drug use – Statistics and facts." November 19. www.statista.com/topics/7786/global-drug-use

Could this widespread struggle be a symptom of a deeper spiritual void? Perhaps it reflects a lack of purpose and meaning in life.

The first self-help group aimed at addressing addiction was Alcoholics Anonymous (AA), founded in Akron, Ohio in 1938. By 1939, AA had published its foundational text, *The Big Book*,[21] and established its first official group at Rockland State Hospital in New York. In 1956, the American Medical Association formally recognized alcoholism as a disease. Today, AA has grown into an international fellowship with over two million members across more than 120,000 groups worldwide (as of 2018).

The principles of AA have been adopted by many other self-help groups over the years:

- Narcotics Anonymous (1953)
- Gamblers Anonymous (1957)
- Overeaters Anonymous (1960)
- Debtors Anonymous (1968)
- Pills Anonymous (1972)
- Workaholics Anonymous (1983)
- Nicotine Anonymous (1982)
- Cancer Anonymous (1987)
- Diabetics Anonymous (1990).

There are also groups for those suffering from:

- phobias (Phobics Anonymous)
- depression (Depressed Anonymous)
- schizophrenia (Schizophrenics Anonymous)
- dual diagnosis disorders (Dual Disorders Anonymous).

Today, 12-step programs are considered an essential part of care for patients with substance use disorders.[22]

Why have these 12-step programs become so popular and widely accepted? The answer may lie in their effectiveness. A comprehensive analysis of 27 studies from

---

21 The book has since been translated into 71 languages, it has large print and abridged versions, and is available in Braille and on cassette, CD, and DVD. In 2019, its 40-millionth copy was printed.

22 Moos, R. and Timko, C. (2008) "Outcome Research on 12-Step and Other Self-Help Programs." In M. Galanter and H. O. Kleber (Eds) *Textbook of Substance Abuse Treatment, 4th edn* (pp.511–521). Washington, DC: American Psychiatric Press.

the Cochrane Library, involving over 10,000 participants, found that AA groups led to higher rates of sustained abstinence compared to other evidence-based treatments such as cognitive behavioral therapy (CBT) or motivational enhancement therapy (MET).[23] Additionally, AA significantly reduced healthcare costs.

AA is often described as "a spiritual program for living." It doesn't require adherence to any specific dogma or creed;[24] instead, it offers a flexible approach to recovery based on spirituality. The program views substance use disorders as diseases affecting not just the body, but also the soul and spirit. The Twelve Steps guide individuals toward spiritual awakening,[25] a process that involves social support, shared beliefs, and a sense of belonging to a community.[26]

This approach seems to help people manage pathological behaviors while developing self-control and coping skills. AA promotes an inclusive form of spirituality that allows members to find their own path—there's no "one-size-fits-all" solution. Instead, participants are encouraged to construct their own spiritual framework as they progress through the 12 steps of the program.

A key aspect of recovery in AA is the willingness to embrace a new way of thinking—a kind of "leap of faith." This involves letting go of self-reliance and trusting in something greater than oneself. For many participants, this shift leads to profound personal transformation.[27]

The success of 12-step programs may also stem from their ability to help people renegotiate their relationship with spirituality in a secular context. As individuals work through the steps, they often experience what AA refers to as "spiritual awakening." This can be sudden or gradual, but is typically marked by feelings of oneness or unity with something larger than oneself—often following periods of intense psychological distress, or "hitting bottom."

Spirituality within AA is closely tied to positive emotions such as awe, love, trust, compassion, gratitude, forgiveness, joy, and hope—all emotions that foster

---

23 "New Cochrane Review finds Alcoholics Anonymous and 12-Step Facilitation programs help people to recover from alcohol problems:" www.cochrane.org/news/new-cochrane-review-finds-alcoholics-anonymous-and-12-step-facilitation-programs-help-people
24 Miller, W. R. and Kurtz, E. (1994) "Models of alcoholism used in treatment: Contrasting AA and other perspectives with which it is often confused." *Journal of Studies on Alcohol* 55, 2, 159–166. doi: 10.15288/jsa.1994.55.159.
25 Dermatis, H. and Galanter, M. (2016) "The role of twelve-step-related spirituality in addiction recovery." *Journal of Religion and Health* 55, 2, 510–521. doi: 10.1007/s10943-015-0019-4.
26 Baker, C. R. (1979) "Defining and measuring affiliation motivation." *European Journal of Social Psychology* 9, 97–99. https://doi.org/10.1002/ejsp.2420090108
27 Kirkland, K. (2018) "The influence of William James on the spirituality of Alcoholics' Anonymous." *Journal of Humanistic Psychology*. www.academia.edu/46501657/The_Influence_of_William_James_on_the_Spirituality_of_Alcoholics_Anonymous

connection with others. These feelings help counteract the isolation often associated with addiction, and can reduce traits such as self-centeredness or egotism,[28] traits that AA identifies as common among addicts.

Hope plays an especially important role in recovery. Many individuals describe addiction as a state of despair where their only faith is placed in drugs or alcohol rather than something higher. Spirituality offers them hope—a belief that things can get better—which motivates them to set goals and strive for more. A systematic review of over 4000 research papers found that factors like supportive social networks, self-efficacy, and having a sense of purpose were all protective against relapse into alcohol use disorder.[29]

According to the World Health Organization's *International Standards for the Treatment of Drug Use Disorders* (2020),[30] one key pillar of recovery is finding resources that allow individuals to rediscover meaning and purpose in life. The spiritual awakening encouraged by 12-step programs may be one such resource—helping people not just recover, but thrive.

Given all this evidence supporting its effectiveness—both spiritually and practically—it's no wonder that recent studies show that 73 percent of substance abuse treatment programs include some form of spirituality-based element in their approach.[31]

MIND–BODY INTERVENTIONS

Mind–body interventions, as defined in Western healthcare and fitness contexts, are practices such as yoga and tai chi that aim to improve physical, mental, and spiritual well-being. The integrative health centers, however, focus on the relationship between the brain, mind, body, environment, and behavior, and how

---

28 Vaillant, G. E. (2013) "Psychiatry, religion, positive emotions and spirituality." *Asian Journal of Psychiatry 6*, 6, 590–594. doi: 10.1016/j.ajp.2013.08.073.
29 Sliedrecht, W., de Waart, R., Witkiewitz, K., and Roozen, H. G. (2019) "Alcohol use disorder relapse factors: A systematic review." *Psychiatry Research 278*, 97–115. https://doi.org/10.1016/j.psychres.2019.05.038
30 WHO (World Health Organization) (2020) *International Standards for the Treatment of Drug Use Disorders*. www.who.int/publications/i/item/international-standards-for-the-treatment-of-drug-use-disorders
31 Grim, B. J. and Grim, M. E. (2019) "Belief, behavior, and belonging: How faith is indispensable in preventing and recovering from substance abuse." *Journal of Religion and Health 58*, 5, 1713–1750. https://doi.org/10.1007/s10943-019-00876-w

they affect both health and disease.[32] While this definition aligns with Western reductionist thought, it often overlooks the deeper layers of these ancient arts. Historically, these practices have been much more than just physical exercises; they've been tools for cultivating mindfulness, tolerance, mutual understanding, increasing awareness, and strengthening the social fabric of entire communities.

Take tai chi, for example. The first written reference to this practice appeared in the *Book of Changes* over 3000 years ago in China. Rooted in Qigong and martial arts traditions, tai chi is a gentle form of exercise where practitioners perform flowing movements while focusing on deep breathing and awareness. It's low impact but powerful in its ability to bring balance to both body and mind.

Yoga has an even longer history. Born in ancient South Asia, its origins can be traced back to the Hindu texts known as the *Vedas*, written around 5000 years ago. Yoga is a group of physical, mental, and spiritual practices aimed at controlling the body and mind to reach enlightenment. In Hinduism, enlightenment is about achieving total awareness—both physically and spiritually—expanding one's consciousness to connect with something greater than oneself.

Historically, these practices have been used not just for physical fitness, but also to promote human flourishing—offering insight into life's deeper questions, fostering peace of mind, and helping individuals connect with a higher purpose while leading to enlightenment.

The health benefits of these practices have been scientifically documented for over 50 years. Early research showed that meditation could reduce oxygen consumption and lower blood pressure—essentially triggering a "relaxation response" that counteracts stress.[33] As interest in these practices grew in the West, so did research into their benefits. Today, we have a wealth of evidence showing how yoga, meditation, and other mind–body therapies can improve both physical health (such as reducing pain) and mental well-being (such as lowering stress).

In fact, mind–body practices are more popular than ever. A recent survey revealed that 14 percent of adults in the US had used techniques like yoga or mindfulness meditation within the past year.[34] Another meta-analysis involving

---

32 Wahbeh, H., Haywood, A., Kaufman, K., and Zwickey, H. (2009) "Mind-body medicine and immune system outcomes: A systematic review." *The Open Complementary Medicine Journal 1*, 25–34. doi: 10.2174/1876391X00901010025.

33 Wallace, R. K., Benson, H., and Wilson, A. F. (1971) "A wakeful hypometabolic physiologic state." *The American Journal of Physiology 221*, 3, 795–799. doi: 10.1152/ajplegacy.1971.221.3.795.

34 Clarke, T. C., Barnes, P. M., Black, L. I., Stussman, B. J., and Nahin, R. L. (2018) "Use of yoga, meditation, and chiropractors among US adults aged 18 and over." NCHS Data Brief No. 325. National Center for Health Statistics, US Centers for Disease Control and Prevention. www.cdc.gov/nchs/products/databriefs/db325.htm?mod=article_inline

over 6400 participants found that these therapies were associated with improved pain management and reduced opioid use—a significant finding given today's opioid crisis.[35]

Although Western medicine has made incredible strides through pharmacotherapies and advanced procedures, it now faces new challenges in tackling stress-related diseases—many of which are linked to lifestyle choices. More Americans than ever are taking prescription medications for chronic conditions caused by stress or poor lifestyle habits. Mind–body therapies offer a helpful complement to traditional treatments by promoting resilience through self-care, practices, and lifestyle changes. While they are not a cure-all, these practices can significantly improve well-being by reducing many of the symptoms of stress-related conditions such as chronic pain or anxiety.

In the next chapter we will examine how the scientific community views spirituality. Although science was originally far removed from spirituality, Paul Mills has discovered otherwise, and describes that "science was originally far removed from spirituality" in his book, *Science, Being, & Becoming: The Spiritual Lives of Scientists*.[36] With quantum physics, the materialistic approach of science has been expanded into unknown possibilities. This, in turn, has opened up some scientists to the fundamental drive of our minds to find the meaning and purpose in our existence, inching them closer to the state of yoga.

---

35   Garland, E. L., Brintz, C. E., Hanley, A. W., Roseen, E. J., *et al*. (2020) "Mind-body therapies for opioid-treated pain: A systematic review and meta-analysis." *JAMA Internal Medicine 180*, 1, 91–105. doi: 10.1001/jamainternmed.2019.4917.

36   Mills, P. J. (Ed.) *Science, Being, & Becoming: The Spiritual Lives of Scientists*. Fort Lauderdale, FL: Light on Light Press.

CHAPTER 4

Towards the State of Yoga

What lies behind us and what lies before us are tiny matters compared to what lies within us.

RALPH WALDO EMERSON (1803–1882)

In previous chapters we considered the current research on spirituality and how it is very much present in our everyday lives. In this chapter we will reflect on what our contemporary scientists and sages say about the mind, consciousness, and self-development.

THE PERSPECTIVE ON CONSCIOUSNESS
Eckhart Tolle says

> the rational mind itself, now so highly developed in the West is the single biggest obstacle to higher consciousness. Thinking has become a disease. Dis-ease happens when things get out of balance. The mind is superb instrument if used rightly. Used wrongly however, it becomes very destructive. You believe that you are your mind. This is a delusion. The instrument has taken you over.[1]

The development of separate individualized ego was perhaps a colossal achievement for human consciousness, but ego has now become the principal obstacle to further human progress.

Scientists are also beginning to talk about the existence of "something more," beyond our material world. Neurosurgeon Eben Alexander writes: "True thought is not the brain's affair. But we have been so trained to associate our brains with

---

1 Tolle, E. (1999) *The Power of Now: A Guide to Spiritual Enlightenment.* Novato, CA: New World Library, p.67.

what we think and who we are that we have lost the ability to realize that we are always much more than our physical brain and physical body."[2] This is the awareness behind the thinking, the Self behind our thought. If we stay at the horizontal level of calculating, judging, and labeling, we won't plug into "something more than our body" very well because we don't really believe it exists. Many of us don't really believe there's anything spiritual beyond this material body. Perhaps those of us in the West have been more strongly influenced by the materialistic worldview more than we realize, but Alexander and other scientists are coming to the recognition that there *is* something more.

QUANTUM PHYSICS MEET ANCIENT WISDOM

Physicist David Bohm[3] postulated that "the thought proceeds as if it is merely reporting objectively, but in fact, it is often coloring and distorting perception in unexpected ways."[4] According to Bohm, "self-awareness is required in order to correct the distortions introduced by thought. Neural receptors throughout the body inform us directly of our physical position and movement. There is no corresponding awareness of the activity of thought. Such an awareness of our thinking process would represent psychological proprioception and would enable the possibility of perceiving and correcting the unintended distortions." As we will see in Chapter 5, examining classical yogic texts, Bohm is indirectly recommending *pratyahara* (the practice of turning inward and detaching from external stimuli*)* and *dharana* (single-object concentration) as introduced by Patanjali's *Yoga Sutras*!

Bohm further proposes that quantum theory implies that elements seemingly separate in space are generally noncausally and nonlocally related projections of a higher dimensional reality. According to Bohm, the physical universe is not all there is, but is only one of many possible orders that could theoretically arise out of the hidden higher dimensional, nonmaterial order. This nonmaterial order continually gives rise, through involution, to the whole space-time, to all creatures within it, including ourselves and to our consciousness as well. This order is

---

2   Alexander, E. (2022) *Proof of Heaven: A Neurosurgeon's Journey into the Afterlife, 10th Anniversary Edition*. New York: Simon & Schuster Paperbacks, p.84.
3   David Joseph Bohm was an American–Brazilian–British scientist, described as one of the most significant theoretical physicists of the 20th century, and who contributed unorthodox ideas to quantum theory, neuropsychology, and the philosophy of mind. He collaborated with Jiddu Krishnamurti for over 25 years, and their recorded dialogues were published in several volumes.
4   Bohm, D. (1994) *Thought as a System*. Oxford: Routledge.

nonmaterial, invisible, but real.[5] Could it possibly be the beginning of the scientific definition of "God"…?

In suggesting a nonmaterial world that gives rise to the physical universe, Bohm is saying what mystics of every major spiritual tradition—Christian, Jewish, Hindu, Buddhist, Muslim, Neoplatonist, and Aboriginal—have been saying for millennia. The world, the mystics say, comes forth from God. Two thousand years ago the philosophy of *Vedanta* declared that material existence was an illusion, a shared dream, from which it was possible to awaken. And when we do, we realize that behind the illusion is pure consciousness. Classical yoga tradition calls it *Ishvara*.

Such unfolding cannot be proven by the "eye" of senses. Nor can it be proven by the intellectual "eye" of the rational mind. The truth of involution can only be seen by one's intuitive vision—through the "eye" of contemplation or meditation. So, if we want to check the truth of unfoldment we need to go deep within to see it. As we will see, Patanjali's *Yoga Sutras* describe a perfect road map to go deep within, to manage the mind, develop its capacity to expand our consciousness, and move us towards the state of yoga.

Amit Goswami,[6] a nuclear physicist, brings quantum paradigm to consciousness and health in his book *The Quantum Doctor*.[7] He suggests that consciousness comes first in healing—it is the ground of all being. Everything else, including matter, is a possibility of consciousness. And consciousness chooses out of these possibilities all the events we experience. In other words, what and how we experience our life depends on the state of our consciousness. That statement is in line with what Marion, Rohr, and Myss postulate.

Goswami further suggests that when medicine is formulated within the integral metaphysics of the primacy of consciousness, conventional (allopathic) medicine and alternative medicine (including the mind–body of Ayurveda and yoga therapy approach) can be reconciled. Not only that, their different domains of applicability, even their interrelationships, are clearly understood.

THE PATH TO HIGHER CONSCIOUSNESS

Conventional medicine or allopathy is based on the premise that disease is due either to external toxic agents such as germs (bacteria and viruses), or to the mechanical malfunctioning of an internal organ of the physical body. In allopathy,

---

5   Bohm, D. (1980) *Wholeness and the Implicate Order*. London and New York: Routledge.
6   https://en.wikiquote.org/wiki/Amit_Goswami
7   Goswami, A. (2011) *The Quantum Doctor: A Quantum Physicist Explains the Healing Power of Integral Medicine*. Charlottesville, VA: Hampton Roads Publishing Company, Inc.

cure is effected mainly by treating the symptoms of the disease until they disappear, via drugs, surgery, or (in the case of cancer) energy radiation.

In contrast, in mind–body medicine, the premise is that disease is due to an imbalance of many factors: the body, mind, spirit, and environment are all interacting in a relationship affecting one another. According to classical yoga (Patanjali's *Yoga Sutras*), the primary cause of illness can be traced to the mind (consciousness). The cure is to correct the problem within the mind so that it will then correct the physiology. This is based on the idea that a nonphysical "life force," variously called subtle energy, *prana*, or chi, is the causal agent behind healing. Subtle energy is not a by-product of material chemistry; instead, it is the movement of a vital world. Hence a more appropriate English word for "subtle" energy is "vital" energy.

From the soul's point of view, the principal purpose of our life here on earth, if not the only purpose, is to grow spiritually, that is, to grow in awareness (expand our consciousness) *by experience*,[8] suggests Marion.

Swami Sivananda Saraswati[9] explains the meaning of yoga:[10]

> many people think that yoga refers to union between body and mind or body, mind and spirit. However, the traditionally accepted meaning is the union between one's individual consciousness and the Universal consciousness. Therefore, yoga refers to a certain state of consciousness (as well as to methods that help one reach that goal), or state of union with the Divine.

TRANSFORMATIONAL JOURNEY THROUGH YOGA

In 2021, in a clinical trial testing psychological mechanisms, Park and her team noted *increased self-transcendence and spiritual peace* as the results produced by yogic practices.[11] Moreover, yoga practice even *without explicit spiritual teachings* can affect the spirituality of individual, as Ness, Briles, and Mellang discovered in 2016.[12] In 2022, Parkinson and Smith confirmed Patanjali's *Yoga Sutras* I:12–14—

---

8   Marion, J. (2004) *The Death of the Mythic God: The Rise of Evolutionary Spirituality*. Charlottesville, VA: Hampton Roads Publishing Company, Inc., p.110.
9   https://en.wikipedia.org/wiki/Sivananda_Saraswati
10 https://sivanandacanada.org/toronto/om
11 Park, C. L., Finkelstein-Fox, L., Groessl, E. J., Elwy, A. R., and Lee, S. Y. (2020) "Exploring how different types of yoga change psychological resources and emotional well-being across a single session." *Complementary Therapies in Medicine* 49, 102354. doi: 10.1016/j.ctim.2020.102354.
12 Ness, A., Briles, K., and Mellan, P. (2016) "Perceptions of yoga spirituality in Minnesota." *Interdisciplinary International Journal* 8, 51–62. https://doi.org/10.36018/dsiij.v8i0.88

the more consistent and the longer the *sadhana*, the more benefits the practitioner achieved.[13]

Such spiritual transformation and expansion of consciousness is very much underestimated by the public as well as many yoga professionals. Yet we also often see it in our clients at our Beyond Cancer retreats.[14] The retreat is residential—clients stay and work together for three weeks in the same small group, which in itself becomes a therapeutic tool. Clients with all cancers at all stages are accepted, providing they can move about independently. Some come within 12 months after finishing treatments. All also come with the severe side effects of chemotherapy and radiation—with high levels of tension, depression, anger, fatigue, and anxiety, as well as chemo brain. Most also have an attitude of victim, which is well entrenched by the healthcare system. Many have never done yoga and do not know what it is about—they just hope it will help them to feel better.

The Beyond Cancer retreat has a very comprehensive protocol, which uses all elements of yoga, not just *asanas*. It takes clients from Day 1 to Day 21 in a systematic way. Yogic techniques are used to work not only on the body, but, more importantly, on emotions and the mind. The aim is to address the causes of the diseases, and not just the symptoms.[15] Clients are helped to recognize carcinogenic thought processes and are given the tools to learn to change their thought patterns and manage their mind. The aim is to help clients resolve or release their negative emotions, which also contribute to the disease and are stored somewhere deep down.

This emphasis, coupled with the intensity of the protocol—six hours per day—and the length of the retreat creates a deep spiritual transformation in many clients. But, most importantly, I believe that the retreats move people—in 21 days—from victimhood to empowerment, helping them to feel "in charge" of their lives. This, in itself, is a tremendous change in life attitude.

How does such radical transformation happen? I guess it has as many ways as there are people. However, here is what we observed at our three-week retreats. Although I describe the process in stages, these may overlap or have a different sequence depending on the individual's spiritual maturity. Most of the clients who

---

13 Parkinson, T. D. and Smith, S. D. (2023) "A cross sectional analysis of yoga experience on variables associated with psychological well-being." *Frontiers in Psychology 13*. doi: 10.3389/fpsyg.2022.999130.
14 Described in Majewski, L. and Bhavanani, A. (2020) *Yoga Therapy as a Whole-Person Approach to Health*. London and Philadelphia, PA: Singing Dragon.
15 Yoga postulates that the dis-ease starts in mental space first—through the unhealthy belief system, negative thoughts, and/or emotions. If not resolved, the abnormality than moves to the subtle energy system (*prana*), creating blocks, and finally manifests as a disease in the physical body.

went through chemotherapy and/or radiation come almost completely disconnected from the body. It has been too excruciating for a long time to feel the side effects of the cancer treatments, so, the first step we work on is reconnection with the body through *asana*, *pranayama*, and increasing proprioception or self-awareness.

Here is the process:

1. *Reconnecting with the body:* As the clients practice, their self-awareness grows and they start feeling subtle energy, manifesting in different sensations within the body. They may feel sudden movement of "some kind of current" or sudden warmth within part or the whole body. They learn to breathe properly, fully engaging the diaphragm. This, in turn, slows down their breathing patterns, thus regulating their nervous system towards a balance between a sympathetic fight/flight response and parasympathetic relaxation response: "Focusing awareness on breath activates all integrative functions of middle pre-frontal cortex. This allows individuals a more objective space from which to be aware of emotions as they arise."[16]

2. *Reconnecting with prana:* As the clients continue to practice, their sensitivity to inner experiences and their curiosity grows. They become more proficient in observing their inner world, and they move towards maintaining the stance of inner witness. Thanks to the brain plasticity, their proprioception grows, and they notice more and more details—not only the body sensation and subtle energy, but now also the emotions rising within.

3. *Observing emotions:* With time and practice, the clients move from "being" emotion into "observing" emotion—from "I am angry" to "I feel anger raising within me." This allows for increased distance to inner experiences, which means they can respond constructively instead of instinctively. As a result, according to interpersonal neurobiology, our emotional stability increases over time. In yoga terms, this is the process of clearing the *kleshas* (psychological distortions) through purification of the *nadis* (subtle energy channels).

4. *Witnessing:* More and more the clients start moving from "doing" to "being," with longer times of parasympathetic relaxation response during the day.

---

16 Parker, S. (2017) *Clearing the Path: The Yoga Way to a Clear & Pleasant Mind: Patanjali, Neuroscience and Emotion*. Minnesota, MN: Ahymsa Publishers, p.161.

The resultant release of oxytocin (the feel-good hormone) into their blood stream relieves their mood problems and counters stress, as well as promoting human bonding and healing—both physical and emotional.

A CASE STUDY IN SPIRITUAL AWAKENING

This progress depends, of course, on each individual's starting point and their level of awareness. On one end of the spectrum we had cancer patients with no body awareness whatsoever and/or with no visualization ability. Their persona was firmly linked with their social role or an idea of their material form. In such cases they were able to gain a very basic connection to their body over the three-week retreat. On the other end of spectrum, we hosted experienced self-aware meditators, who were able to experience significant shifts in their level of consciousness. They arrived at the retreat already reconnected with their body and emotions, perhaps not yet fully settled in their witness, but having tasted it from time to time.

In both cases, the intensity of yogic practices in a small group would bring forward unresolved issues in the clients' relationships with others and with themselves. This was fascinating to watch as the presence of others always seemed to intensify the process of cleansing. The group would become a catalyst and at the same time, paradoxically, a very strong supportive factor helping individuals face their unresolved issues. Clients would also move from a false identity, such as "I am"—a parent, a partner, an engineer, a yoga teacher, a therapist—towards witness identity. From a superficial role identity to spiritual presence identity.

Consequently, the change in their level of consciousness would alter their mind field from what Stephen (Stoma) Parker calls a weaker to stronger mind field.[17] As a result, the clients would change their outlook on life and their attitudes:

- From demanding to giving
- From judging to accepting
- From seeking pleasure to taking joy in the pleasure of others
- From indulging (to fill emptiness) to a sense of inner fullness and contentment
- From speaking loudly to be heard to speaking softly, from inner silence
- From seeking attention to influencing through presence

---

17 Parker, S. (2017) *Clearing the Path: The Yoga Way to a Clear & Pleasant Mind: Patanjali, Neuroscience and Emotion*. Minnesota, MN: Ahymsa Publishers, p.227.

- From moving randomly to moving with grace and economy
- From easily distracted to focused and concentrated
- From feeling lonely when alone to feeling solitary, by oneself, with oneself
- From rigidity in beliefs and behavior to flexibility of thought and emotion
- From justification of behavior to apology for the action
- From holding a grudge to forgiving and moving on
- From blaming self and others to taking responsibility.

Needless to say, a stronger mind may result in much a happier and more useful life. I must also add a caveat here—oftentimes we, as facilitators, didn't realize the end impact of the retreat on our clients. Some can feel the difference as they leave for home, as the following client stated:

> I am so glad I found this course and was able to come. It's exactly what I needed at this point in my cancer recovery. I came into this course feeling depressed, hopeless, fatigued, and disconnected from my body. I am now leaving three weeks later with a sense of hope for a meaningful and rich life, a feeling of joy returning and with greater energy and belief in my body.

Clients, often, however, did not realize the depth of their inner transformation. They were only able to appreciate the inner changes when returning to their home environment. Such was the case with Nick P., a 72-year-old psychotherapist from England, who had never practiced yoga before and who knew very little about it. He also considered himself to be a sworn atheist. Here we quote verbatim, with his permission, the story as he wrote it about six months after attending the retreat.

> I had decided to attend the three-week course in October 2014 run by Lee Majewski at Kaivalydham Yoga Institute in India, south east of Mumbai, as I was recovering from some severe arthritis following a period of feeling really unwell after food poisoning in Sri Lanka. Well, that was one demonstrable symptom but perhaps also, just getting older was another, having passed my 72nd birthday and deeply conscious that for the last lap of this race we all run, I needed to pay closer attention to my body and to my mind. I had at that stage not really thought about my heart.
>   The course was a daily program of very gentle yoga postures, *pranayama* breath routines, awareness, study, and chanting, not to mention lovely simple food, day after day. A nice cocktail! The first week is, of course, always the

hardest, and I duly struggled while at the same time noting an almost immediate increase in general vitality, which I ascribed to *pranayama*. Looking back on the experience I now see just how deeply significant and necessary this practice of breath work really is. I had for years tried to meditate, but it was not really until I started working with the breath that I realized that to watch the breath is to meditate.

The second week seems to be the week when "the stuff rises," so to speak, and in my case this was most certainly the case. It took the form of finding myself almost uncontrollably angry at our course leader...poor Lee. This exploded one day and I attacked her verbally, an assault in the face of which she stood calmly firm and looked at me with increased attention. We subsequently had a chat about it and I realized I was projecting an old hatred born of fear onto her, and having seen it, as is the way with these things...it collapsed and I was free of it, important in what was to happen next.

Kindly, I think partly as a result of this, Lee started in our meditation sessions to direct us to working on the heart center (heart chakra, as it's called in the Indian Tradition). This, for me, was the crowning experience of my whole visit, and I came to realize just how helpful the whole chakra system really is in helping us to unblock old wounds. I suppose I have here to own that, on reflection, in spite of many attempts to be otherwise, my heart still remained closed. This is a terrible condition and one I suspect very common in the West, for if the heart is closed, then "loving" is not really possible. We may seek "love" as hard as we like, but "loving," loving life, loving people, loving all experience, eludes us. A most painful condition that arises I suspect from very early birth or childhood traumatic experience in which the heart closes in order to survive. And when the heart closes out of these traumatic contacts with the world, it builds around itself a hard casing like an old walnut that has sat beside the fire all winter. Hard and very difficult to crack open.

Working with the heart center for us meant repeatedly bringing our attention to bear on the heart, imaginary breathing in and out of the heart, evoking in the heart positive emotions such as gratefulness, kindness, appreciation, mercy, and finally perhaps love itself. When I commenced this I have to say I was a bit suspicious. Was this just a new age dream? Did it actually do anything?

In one session quietly concentrating on my heart it suddenly burst into flame. I could not believe it; I suddenly had a veritable bonfire going in the area of the heart. Small to begin with, it began to flower until my whole interior horizon was ablaze. The session finished and I was left dumb with wondering, weepy, slightly shaken, unsure of what had happened but realizing something big really had happened. We dispersed for lunch and I wandered off on my own towards the kitchens.

As I entered the courtyard a clear intuition came over me that I had not quite finished this piece of work and so, seeking out a chair under a tree, I re-entered my interior world and brought my attention back to the fire in my heart. Almost immediately I saw the fire glowing deep down inside me and my attention was taken by one small specific coal that seemed to glow more brightly than the others. In my imagination I picked this glowing coal up in my fingers and stared at it deeply. In a flash I immediately vanished deep, deep inside myself, deeper than in any meditation I had ever done before, and I swam around inside myself like this for some minutes, head "deep under water," so to speak. I suddenly popped out again and went and had lunch!

This experience stayed with me when I returned to the UK, and it's as if a whole new dimension has arisen in my experience of being alive. I find it the most potent antidote to negative feelings and emotions. Should these crowd in upon me (as they want to do in grey old January London!?) I simply bring my attention to the heart and circle around it with positive affirmations of emotions such as joy, loving gratefulness for what I have, rather than what I do not have, and lo and behold my negative feelings evaporate. As I usually do this in the early morning I come down to breakfast and my wife says, "Why are you so damn cheerful?"

Also I think once we re-open this center in ourselves, a compulsion seems to arise, and it certainly did in me, to be more honest with ourselves and more straightforward and honest with others. I found myself being much more critical of myself in terms of relationships, wanting things straightforward, nothing concealed, a higher integrity, as if the heart could not stand anything not quite right, not straight and authentic. Finally, it seemed to me as if one other essential faculty was restored to me through this heart center work, and that was that my gratefulness heart meditations turned into what I can only describe as praise. This did not seem to be praise to a specific God, or even an idea like it, but to something out and beyond my small self, something altogether larger and more powerful than myself, to which the only right attitude seemed to be praise. This has given my life a new sense of direction in this respect, and it is a joyful thing.

So, having completed this retreat and having been able to keep my practice going on my return to England, my advice would be, chuck the antidepressants away, stop rushing around trying to distract yourself with ever finer distractions, breathe, meditate, and bring your attention to the heart again and again, until it fills you up. You may be surprised!

Namaste.

Nick P.

THE PATH TO A STATE OF YOGA

This dramatic spiritual transformation opened "a whole new dimension…in the experience of being alive" for our client, changing his attitude towards life and "wanting things straightforward, nothing concealed, a higher integrity as if the heart could not stand anything not quite right, not straight and authentic." Although an atheist, Nick P. suddenly found something more—"something out and beyond my small self, something altogether larger and more powerful than myself, to whom the only right attitude seemed to be praise. This has given my life a new sense of direction in this respect, and it is a joyful thing."

This experience motivated Nick P. after going back home to dive deep into studying yoga, and especially Patanjali's *Yoga Sutras*. A few years later he wrote to me:

> I run study groups now on Patanjali because I think he, more than anyone else I know, articulates so well the difference between psychical and spiritual. The intense priority is to get ourselves free from psychical enmeshment *then* we begin to get an idea of how it actually binds us and *how* we can become freer. Good psychotherapy! It seems to me this is the best way to deal with the various demons hanging on to our toes so we may get a glimpse of what the spiritual is…we do so love to take short cuts!

Was it a gateway to Dr. Miller's awakened awareness? A shift to Marion's next level of consciousness? We don't know. However, we do know that the extended length and intensity of yogic practices created a profound spiritual shift in Nick P. and in many other clients. It left them with profound changes in their world view, which now included something bigger than their small self. It also made them much happier and more peaceful human beings—it brought them closer to the state of yoga.

In the next chapter we'll dive deeper into understanding yoga's true depth—and how its spiritual aspects can help eradicate suffering from our and our clients' lives.

CHAPTER 5

Spirituality in Classical Yogic Texts

Connect with Higher Consciousness daily!
BHAGAVAD GITA, CHAPTER 6 (2ND OR 1ST CENTURY BCE)

We will start with a few words on the history of a general understanding of health:

> The concept of health as a balance between a person and the environment, the unity of soul and body, and the natural origin of disease, was the backbone of the perception of health in ancient Greece. Similar concepts existed in ancient Indian known as Ayurveda. Ayur in Sanskrit means life, veda means knowledge, thus Ayurveda translates to knowledge (science) of life.[1]

In the 5th century BC, Pindar defined health as a "harmonious functioning of the organs," emphasizing the physical dimension of health, the physical body, and overall functionality, accompanied by the feeling of comfort and absence of pain. Even today, his definition bears importance as a prerequisite for overall health and wellness.

Plato (429–347 BC), in his *Dialogues*, pointed out that a perfect human society could be achieved by harmonizing the interests of the individual and the community, and that the ideal of ancient Greek philosophy—"a healthy mind in a healthy body"—could be achieved if people established internal harmony and harmony with the physical and social environment. Aristotle (384–322 BC) emphasized the necessity for regulating relations in society to achieve harmonious functioning

---

[1] Svalastog, A. L., Donev, D., Kristoffersen, N. J., and Gajović, S. (2017) "Concepts and definitions of health and health-related values in the knowledge landscapes of the digital society." *Croatian Medical Journal 58*, 6, 431–435. https://doi.org/10.3325/cmj.2017.58.431

and preserving the health of its members. Hippocrates (460–c. 370 BC) explained health in connection with environmental factors and lifestyle. He was the creator of the concept of "positive health," which depended on the primary human constitution (which we consider today as genetics), diet, and exercise.

Today, all modern concepts of health recognize it as something more than the absence of disease, implying a maximum capacity of the individual for self-realization and self-fulfillment. The World Health Organization's (WHO) definition from 1946 states: "Health is a state of complete physical, mental and social well-being and not merely the absence of disease or infirmity."[2] With growing social awareness in the last few decades, several attempts have been made to amend this definition with a fourth dimension, "spiritual health," albeit to date unsuccessfully.

There are also different approaches to health today. Conventional allopathic medicine deals mainly with the body as a sum of organs and focuses on the factors that cause the disease—which is a pathogenetic approach. Ayurveda, Traditional Chinese Medicine, and yoga therapy take a different view and focus on what creates health and the factors supporting health—this is the theory of salutogenesis.

As we will see in this chapter, the traditional yogic texts promise to ward off disease and improve health and well-being, providing we properly abide by the rules and regulations (*Hathapradipika* I:64). In another classical text the human body is likened to an unbaked clay pot. It is only through the practice of yoga that the human body is baked, making it fit to hold Divine Spirit (*Gheranda Samhita* I:8). We described this in more detail in our book, *Yoga Therapy as a Whole-Person Approach to Health*.[3]

The focus of yoga practices is on cleansing the *nadis* (energetic channels). Through this experiential process, we connect to our own Spirit, thus unveiling our connection to a Higher Power/God/Universal Consciousness and achieving the state of yoga, unity with the transcendental. Health and well-being are created when our Spiritual Being is integrated with our physical, energetic, emotional, and mental bodies all in balance. The use of yoga therapy is just a recent happening, a profession in the making. In its wonderfully long history yoga served to promote our spiritual evolution. Even so, the traditional texts are full of reference to specific practices bringing balance to the three humors

---

2   www.who.int/about/governance/constitution
3   Majewski, L. and Bhavanani, A. (2020) *Yoga Therapy as a Whole-Person Approach to Health*. London and Philadelphia, PA: Singing Dragon.

(*vata*, *pitta*, *kapha*), and thus restoring health according to the theory of health developed in the late Vedic era.

One of the foremost concepts of yoga therapy is that the mind influences the body (and vice versa), thus creating disease or health. This is the basis for psychosomatics and mind–body medicine. In modern language it is termed psycho-neuro-immunology. Today, even modern allopathic health systems have realized the importance of the placebo effect and how the content of what we think and how we feel influences our nervous, endocrine, and immune responses.

Unlike allopathic medicine, the yogic concept of health and disease has its source not in the body but through blockages in our subtler energy system. All disturbances start at the psychic level, beyond the mind (the psyche in Indian thought goes all the way up to the sense of Self). If not resolved they come down through the disturbed mind, and then manifest in subtle energy channels (*prana nadi*), and finally settle in the physical body, manifesting as the disease of the body.

While the modern allopathic medical model mostly deals with this last layer—the physical body—yoga therapy looks for the root cause of the manifested disease in the five-layered model of human existence (the *pancha koshas* system). The allopathic model also looks at the disease (a pathogenetic approach), which manifests in the body or mind. Yoga therapy seeks the balance and coherence of all layers of human existence,[4] as per the three *doshas* (energy patterns) (*vata*, *pitta*, *kapha*), the *pancha koshas* (five sheaths or layers) (*annamaya*, the physical body; *pranamaya*, the energy body; *manomaya*, the mental body; *vijnanamaya*, the intellectual body; and *anandamaya*, the bliss body), the *gunas* (qualities) (*sattva*, *rajas*, *tamas*), and the *pancha vayus*.

While in Western culture the definition and understanding of spirituality is still evolving, we—yoga teachers and therapists—are lucky to have classical yogic texts. As we explore these texts, we will find that they offer a wonderful road map to spirituality and to the development of awakened awareness in each of us. Contrary to the popular belief in the West that yoga equals an *asana* class consisting of strange body postures, traditional yogic texts speak to much deeper dimensions of yoga, which some may not appreciate. Yoga philosophy and ancient texts, such as Patanjali's *Yoga Sutras* and *Hathapradipika*, offer deep understanding of spirituality as a source of health—the connection that Western researchers only now seem to be rediscovering. These texts, as we will see, also offer the way to achieve such health.

---

4   We elaborate on this more in Majewski, L. and Bhavanani, A. (2020) *Yoga Therapy as a Whole-Person Approach to Health*. London and Philadelphia, PA: Singing Dragon.

Health in Sanskrit is *svastha*. *Hathapradipika* in IV:112 defines *svastha* as the state of liberation—a state in which a person is so deep within themselves and aware of their inner world that they perceive it but are not moved by any outside object or relationship. If we look at the etymology of the word, the connection to health becomes clearer. Patanjali's *Yoga Sutras* in 2:23 uses *sva* to mean individual "Self," while *stha* means "stay." It can be understood as *"I am healthy if I stay connected to my Self."*

On the other hand, *vyadhi*, as per Patanjali's *Yoga Sutras*, means disease, one of nine obstacles in the path of yogic practices. *Vi* stands for disconnection and *adi* means something deeper within an individual. We can understand this to mean *"When I am disconnected from my inner Self, I am diseased."* So even this ancient language points us to the way towards health.

Most of us are taught to live our life with our antennas directed exclusively to the outside world, often not being aware of what is happening inside us. We care what others think of us, what image we project, how many possessions we have, and how others perceive us. In addition, those who suffer chronic pain or chronic disease often tend to disconnect from their body on purpose, so that they do not feel the pain or discomfort of chronic disease.

And yet, our body repeatedly reveals to us what is going on inside us. Our bodies react to the environment and hold the memories of unresolved issues from the past. Our emotions, of which we are frequently not aware, make us react instinctively, without forethought. Our thoughts run rampant, ruminating, and we tend to run, catching life on the go, just like we grab a cup of coffee to go. We identify with our bodies, trying to make them perfect, or we identify with our thoughts, not really knowing who we truly are. As enlightened masters say—we are walking in our sleep, totally unaware of our own inner world. No wonder chronic diseases are so predominant today.

The challenges of modern life often leave us feeling disconnected from the natural flow of existence. As we rush through the various stages of life, it's easy to feel unsettled or adrift, unsure of our roles, responsibilities, and purpose. This sense of disconnection is often compounded by societal pressures, where we are driven by material success, personal achievements, and external validations. Consequently, it's not uncommon for people to feel unfulfilled at various stages of life, uncertain about what is expected of them, and unsure of how to transition smoothly into the next phase.

THE FOUR *ASHRAMAS*: ANCIENT WISDOM FOR MODERN LIFE

In the ancient Vedic tradition,[5] the four *ashramas*, or stages of life, provided a clear and structured path designed to guide individuals through the various phases of human existence. These stages—called *brahmacharya* (student of life), *grihastha* (householder stage of life), *vanaprastha* (retirement), and *sannyasa* (life of renunciation)—offered a framework for living a balanced, purposeful life, founded on spiritual and ethical principles.

Each stage had its own set of duties and responsibilities, which were aligned with the natural progression of life. By adhering to this structure, individuals could live in harmony with their surroundings and with themselves. Although these stages were outlined thousands of years ago, the underlying wisdom remains deeply relevant today, especially as many of us grapple with questions of purpose, fulfillment, and identity.

Let's take a closer look at these four stages, and consider how they can offer guidance for navigating the complexities of modern life.

Brahmacharya ashrama (student of life)

The *brahmacharya* stage, which spans the early years of life (approximately the first 25 years), is a time of education and self-discipline. Ancient yogis believed that this stage was critical for laying the foundations for a life of purpose, virtue, and knowledge. During this period, individuals were expected to cultivate self-control, simplicity, and a deep sense of respect for their teachers and elders. The emphasis was on learning, both academically and spiritually, and preparing oneself for the responsibilities that would come in later life.

In today's world, the *brahmacharya* stage can be seen as a time for young people to explore their interests, develop their skills, and build character. While modern education often focuses on academic achievement, the wisdom of the *Vedas* claims that true learning goes beyond textbooks. It encompasses moral education, life skills, and the ability to navigate challenges with grace and resilience. Practicing yoga during this stage can help young people develop self-awareness, emotional intelligence, and a sense of balance—qualities that are essential for a fulfilling life.

---

5 The *Veda* is a collection of poems or hymns composed in archaic Sanskrit by Indo-European-speaking peoples who lived in northwest India during the 2nd millennium BCE. There were four *Vedas*: *Rigveda* (1500–1200 BCE), and *Yajurveda*, *Samaveda*, and *Atharvaveda* (1200–900 BCE).

Grihastha ashrama (householder stage life)

The *grihastha* stage, which spans the middle years of life (approximately 25–50 years), is often the most active and demanding phase. This is the time when individuals take on the responsibilities of family life, marriage, a career, and contributing to society. In the Vedic tradition, marriage was seen not just as a social contract but as a sacred union aimed at personal and spiritual growth. The responsibilities of this stage, such as raising children and managing a household, were viewed as opportunities for spiritual development.

In modern times, the *grihastha* stage is often associated with the pressures of career advancement, financial responsibilities, and social obligations. Yet, the ancient yogis taught, this stage does not have to be merely about material success. By approaching our duties with mindfulness and a spirit of service, it is possible to transform even the most mundane tasks into opportunities for growth and fulfillment. Yoga can be a powerful tool during this stage, helping individuals cultivate inner peace amidst the busyness of life, reminding them of the deeper purpose behind their daily actions.

Vanaprastha ashrama (retirement)

The *vanaprastha* stage, which begins around the age of 50, marks a transition from the active responsibilities of the householder to a more contemplative and introspective phase of life. In ancient times, this was a period when individuals would withdraw from the hustle of worldly life and devote themselves to social service, mentorship, and spiritual practice. The idea was not to detach completely from society, but to shift focus from personal gains to the welfare of others.

In today's world, retirement is often viewed as the end of our productive life, which can lead to feelings of isolation, boredom, or a loss of purpose. However, the wisdom of the *vanaprastha* stage encourages us to see this phase as an opportunity for renewal and growth. Rather than retreating from life, those in the *vanaprastha* stage could take on the role of mentors, offering their wisdom and experience to younger generations. Yoga can play a vital role in this stage, helping individuals maintain physical vitality, mental clarity, and spiritual connection as they navigate the challenges of aging.

Sannyasa ashrama (life of renunciation)

The final stage, *sannyasa*, is one of complete renunciation. In this stage, individuals are no longer bound by worldly attachments and are free to pursue spiritual enlightenment. The *sannyasi* is a seeker of truth, focused on the ultimate purpose of life—the realization of the Self and the union with the Universal Consciousness.

This stage represents the culmination of our spiritual journey, where the individual transcends the ego and lives in a state of pure awareness.

While few people in the modern world may choose to embark on a formal path of renunciation, the essence of *sannyasa* can still be experienced. As we age, many of us naturally begin to let go of material attachments, seeking deeper meaning in life. Yoga, with its emphasis on self-realization and inner peace, can guide us through this process, helping us cultivate a sense of detachment, acceptance, and spiritual fulfillment.

Contrary to the previous stages, motivation in *sannyasa* was pure, the individual was disinterested in the fruits of the action. The action came from a sense of duty or a command that came from the conscience without thinking about gains or losses, maybe even at the cost of their life. Only a *sannyasi* would be motivated to perform an action without attachment to the result. The simple dress of a *sannyasi* symbolized the ideal of life for which the individual stood and lived. A *sannyasi* surrendered their home and possessions because they perceived the whole Universe as their home. They were above fears, passions, and hatred. They were free from likes and dislikes, desires, egoism, lust, anger, greed, and pride. They were true yogis!

It's true that the world we live in today is vastly different from the one in which the *Vedas* were written. In the West especially, the pace of life is often frantic, marriages are increasingly viewed as temporary contracts, and elders are frequently marginalized or isolated in retirement homes. The result is an increasing sense of loneliness and disconnection, which many people feel at various stages of their lives. However, as we see in the growing popularity of yoga, there is a deep, collective yearning for the values that the ancient yogis espoused—simplicity, purity, hard work, devotion to knowledge, and spiritual growth. People who practice yoga regularly often find themselves naturally gravitating towards these principles, even if they initially came to yoga for physical fitness or stress relief. Over time, the practice begins to transform not just the body, but the mind, the emotions, and spirit as well.

Curious minds may ask, how does this transformation happen? Let us examine two of the most famous classical yogic texts—Patanjali's *Yoga Sutras* and *Hathapradipika*—to find the answer to this question.

PATANJALI'S *YOGA SUTRAS*

Perhaps we can find the answers in Patanjali's *Yoga Sutras*, 196 short aphorisms, which were transmitted by oral tradition around 1000 BC and then written down by Patanjali some time around 500 BC–300 AD. Divided into four *padas* (chapters), they explain the goal of yoga and the means to achieve it. They need to be studied closely to grasp the depth of their meaning. As one of my clients, a psychotherapist, has said, these *sutras* are the best psychotherapy guidance in the world.

We encourage readers who have a basic idea about the practice of yoga but who do not know the *Yoga Sutras* to read and contemplate the deeper meaning of these *sutras*. It is not within the scope of this book to analyze each *sutra* as many excellent translations and expositions already exist. We will only describe the main points in general terms as they pertain to spirituality and are important to yoga professionals and answer our question about transformative power.

Samadhi pada

In the first *pada*, Patanjali describes the goal of yoga and possible obstacles in achieving it. Against common understanding within the Western yoga community today, the goal of yoga is not self-regulation or relaxation. At the very beginning Patanjali points to the goal of yoga as the process of mental purification and the expansion of consciousness.

Jim Marion's nine stages of consciousness begs the question—can such purification and expansion of consciousness result in moving from one stage of consciousness to a higher one? My answer to that is—*yes*! In our three-week Beyond Cancer healing retreats, where clients performed six hours of yoga for 20 days, we witnessed spiritual transformation to a certain degree in almost everyone, resulting in a changed approach to life as well to their own health. Oftentimes it manifested in miraculous transformation of personality and attitudes as well as understanding their purpose in life.

Explanation for such a transformation comes in the following *sutra*: "this allows one to reconnect and establish one's identity within one's own *Atman*/Self/Consciousness" (Patanjali's *Yoga Sutras* 1:1–4). By definition, then, the *Yoga Sutras* point us to spiritual journey within, to coming Home to Self. Such a journey is brought by sustained yogic practices, performed continuously for a long time with reverence and careful attention, and by discernment or dispassionate objectivity (Patanjali's *Yoga Sutras* 1:12–14).

As we practice yoga we travel, knowingly or unknowingly, on the spiritual path that leads to recognition that our current perception of reality, of the world and of others, is skewed by our acquired and innate conditioning (*samskaras*).

Consequently, we begin to realize that our perception of the world around us is distorted by our own subjective experiences and psychological development. Patanjali calls this *avidya*, innate ignorance. With time and yogic practices, we increase the awareness of our own ignorance and conditioning, and our view of ourselves and the world changes. Our consciousness expands.

Patanjali then stresses that the state of yoga is brought by the union between Self (*atman*) and the Divine (*Ishvara*). The time that is required to overcome obstacles and achieve a yoga state depends on us and our intensity, zeal, enthusiasm, energy, and sincerity in performing our yogic *sadhana* (yogic practices). Because the wisdom gained through yoga is *experiential*, reading about it or debating it doesn't do anything.

This, perhaps, is the most important point that needs to be stressed. In our education we are used to learning intellectually. We read, memorize facts, and debate ideas. This is all important, yet in yoga it is even more important to maintain daily yogic practices with intention and attention. These practices have the transformational power to change us in many ways— physical, energetic, emotional, mental, and spiritual.

Patanjali defines the Divine (*Ishvara*) as a unique indwelling, unchanging Omnipresence, existing within each one of us. It is That (which cannot be named) which is left over when the ego and ignorance collapses. It is also described as a canvas on which our life experiences appear, an Omniscience or inner intelligence that is unconditioned by time or experiences. It is our Soul/Self. This makes yoga accepting and universally applicable to all religions. The verbal representation of the Divine is *Pranava*, the mantra "OHM." When chanted in a sustained manner it turns the awareness within, and dispels the distractions and obstacles, allowing for saturation of the whole being with Divine Intelligence (1:23–29).

The stronger our *sadhana*, with intent (*sankalpa*) and sustained effort, the less grip our psychological conditioning (*kleshas*) has on us has us, and the closer to the Divine Intelligence or Light within we get. The closer to the Divine we get, the easier it is for us to submit our ego to the Divine and hear Its guidance. This way the *sadhana* completely transforms our entire being and there is a total change of personality, understanding of life, and of our purpose. All habits and tendencies are overcome by such habitual self-awareness (1:40–51)!

Patanjali also cautions us about many internal obstacles in performing our *sadhana* (1:30–39). Illness, indecision, procrastination, sloth, sensual craving, inability to maintain the state achieved earlier—these obstacles may manifest as pain or suffering, depression, and irregular breathing, among others.

Patanjali then goes on to suggest different methods in preventing and dealing with these obstacles. Perhaps the most important is to choose the practices of one lineage and to stay with those, rather than moving around different lineages indiscriminately, without achieving or experiencing the depth of the practice.

In a nutshell, in the first *pada* Patanjali describes in detail the goal of yoga as achieving the deep spiritual transformation of the practitioner towards a higher level of consciousness. He also stresses that reading about it and taking it in intellectually will not produce good results. This is *experiential* endeavor—we must practice daily, with inner discipline, one-pointedness and dedication, in order to reap the benefits and attain the promises contained in this text.

Sadhana pada

In the second and third *padas* Patanjali describes in general terms the road map leading to achieving the goal outlined in the first *pada*. The second *pada* explains the importance of *sadhana* (sustained daily yoga practice) as a step-by-step journey to a higher state of consciousness—remember Marion's states of consciousness!

Patanjali starts with recommending the three-prong *Kriya Yoga* practice (2:1), which brings a lessening of the *kleshas* (psychological distortions). These are:

- Austerity (*tapas*) as an attitude towards one's physical and physiological needs
- The study of sacred texts, recitation of mantras, and self-introspection (*svadhyaya*)
- Devotion to *Ishvara*, ability to surrender to Divine will and let go of the end goal (*Ishvara pranidhana*).

Patanjali then proceeds with explaining the five psychological distortions (*kleshas*), which most humans have to deal with (2:3–9):

- Ignorance, which makes us believe that the reality we see is the ultimate, seeing the impure to be pure, the suffering to be pleasure, and the non-self to be Self (*avidya*)
- Egoism, resulting from identifying with our body, our mind, or ego instead of Self (*asmita*)
- Attraction to that which is pleasurable (*raga*)
- Aversion to that which gives us pain or suffering (*dwesha*)
- A basic survival instinct caused by fear of death (*abhinivesha*).

Patanjali then proceeds to describe the ways of removing these afflictions as the process of purification of the body, mind, and spirit, resulting in expansion of our consciousness. In this process the practitioner (*sadhaka*) unveils the Divinity within, the Self, enabling access to the highest Wisdom (2:28). As a road map to achieving this, Patanjali presents the eight limbs (*angas*) of yoga, also called *Ashtanga* or *Raja Yoga* (2:29–55). The first five *angas* called, external (*biharanga*) yoga, deal with our body vs. the external world:

- Code of ethics in social conduct: *yama*
- Code of inner conduct: *niyama*
- Body postures that bring physical equilibrium: *asana*
- Breathing techniques that bring mental equilibrium: *pranayama*
- Beginning of the management of the senses and focusing of the mind: *pratyahara*.

Today, it seems that *yama* and *niyama* have almost been forgotten in Western yoga circles. Yet, as a code of conduct, these two should be guiding our intentions and actions, guiding our daily life. There is also an inherent promise of attainment of some *siddhis* (extraordinary psychic abilities) when a certain degree of perfection is reached in the respective *yama* and *niyama*.

The five *yamas* are moral restraints that cultivate control over our lower human tendencies:

- Nonviolence, which includes the mental, physical, or psychological aspects of attitudes towards ourself and others. In other words, abstaining from injuring any being at any time in any manner (2:35): *ahimsa*.

- Truthfulness at all times. This means the effort to make the mind and speech correspond to the thing that has been correctly comprehended, walking the talk (2:36): *satya*.

- Nonstealing, whether physical, mental, or psychological—abstaining from desiring and/or unlawfully taking things belonging to others (2:37): *asteya*.

- Control of creative energies within, as well as managing urges of a sexual nature and managing the organs that lead to sexual excitement. Thinking of, talking about, joking, looking intently, secret talk, resolve, attempt, and execution are the eight forms of sexual indulgence, say the sages. The yogi should practice their opposites (2:38): *brahmacharya*.

- Nonpossessiveness, noncontrolling—as the yogi seeks selflessness in realization, it is inevitable for them to give up completely all objects of enjoyment (2:39): *aparigraha*.

Five *niyamas* are ethical observances that cultivate humane qualities, preparing us for the conscious life in yoga:

- Cleanliness at all levels: mental, emotional, and physical. It is necessary for the yogi to keep their mind and body clean. The place of residence should be clean and the food intake only pure. Through internal purification the yogi cleanses the mind of impurities such as arrogance, conceit, malice, etc. (2:40–41): *shaucha*.

- Self-contentment may result in attaining happiness; the gratitude for "What I have is enough" should be cultivated and meditated upon (2:42): *santosha*.

- Self-discipline, the ability to maintain constant effort, the endurance of the body and mind should be practiced through the observance of austerities. When the body develops the power to endure hardship and when the mind does not get easily upset, we become qualified on the path of yoga (2:43): *tapas*.

- Self-introspection, self-observance, self-awareness—through the study of yogic texts, worldly thoughts decrease and instead the taste for the spiritual path prevails (II:44): *swadhyaya*.

- Letting go of ego and letting in the Divine will—through giving up the desired fruit of the actions we are able to completely surrender to the Divine. By meditating on the Divine as Consciousness within the Self, the yogi realizes their own individual Self/Divinity (2:45): *Ishwara pranidhana*.

Patanjali also presents the concept *pratipaksha bhavana* (2:33), consisting of replacing any negative or destructive thought or attitude with its opposite, the positive one. It is the original cognitive behavioral therapy (CBT)! I find it a very useful tool to manage my mind in everyday life. Anytime I notice my mind goes into a negative or destructive spin, I simply say "Cancel, cancel," and direct my mind towards a different subject.

The next yoga *anga* is *asana*. Unfortunately, *asana* seems to still be the most predominantly used as the synonym of yoga. Yet, out of 196 *Yoga Sutras*, only three are dedicated to *asana* (2:46–48), which is less then 1.2 percent of the whole of yoga!! *Asana* is described as a state that radiates stability and ease, and is to be practiced with relaxation, self-awareness, and contemplation of the infinite. Practicing *asana* this way results in balanced equanimity, of mind, emotions, and body, promises Patanjali.

Pranayama (2:49–53)—the next *anga*—is the management of life force (*prana*) through exhalation, inhalation, and suspension of the breath. Patanjali describes *pranayama* as a bridge between the external and internal world, detailing different practices through which the mind prepares for the next *anga*. This is where the transition from external to internal yoga begins. It is often said that *pranayama* is the bridge between the body and the mind.

Pratyahara (2:54–55) is the last of external yoga, and regarded by some as the beginning of inner (*antaranga*) yoga. It is the process of active withdrawing of the mind at will from the sensory engagement with outside reality. With the help of *pranayama*, we withdraw our mind from the external world, focusing it on our breath—our inner world. This is a transition from focusing on our body in relation to the outside world, to turning our awareness towards the content of the mind. This is why the next three *angas* of Patanjali's *Yoga Sutras* are called "inner" (*antaranga*) yoga.

Vibhuti pada

We know that we cannot see beyond our own limited vision. To evolve this vision from the level of the material world into higher realms of perception we must go through the process of mental training—a process of intense concentration. The process of training of the mind started with *pratyahara*, when we were learning to withdraw our attention from our senses, of what we hear, smell, taste, and feel in the body. We close our eyes to shut out visual input from the outer world.

The third *anga*—*vibhuti pada*—is all about the next stages of gradually training our mind. They come in the stages of *dharana*, *dhyana*, and *samadhi*. As we continue our daily practice of *pratyahara*, the ability to hold focus in one place or point for a long time increases. In this process there are still three distinct factors:

1. There is an observer
2. There is the observed
3. There is a process of observation.

As the practitioner holds the focus on the object, they are fully aware of time and space and the distinction between these three factors—of themselves as a subject, the object of observation, and the fact that they are observing. This stage is called *dharana*.

With time and sustained practice, we lose the sense of ourself, and the observer becomes one with the observed, losing awareness of the process of observation. How long we have to practice to reach this stage depends on our individual level of awareness and level of consciousness, as each of us is different. When all three factors fold into one, we lose awareness of the body and mind. There is nothing but meditative experience, and that state Patanjali calls *dhyana*, or meditation.

For example, we focus on the flower and are able to hold the flower in our mind for a particular period of time. However, we are not able to forget about ourselves. We are still aware of time and space. This is *dharana*. When we are able to hold the concept of the flower in our mind, there is no sense of an observation process, and we are no longer aware of ourselves—this is *dhyana*.

When we are able to hold the concept of the flower in our mind and the flower within becomes a living experience so that there is no difference between the external flower (experience) and internal flower (experience) and they look alike, Patanjali calls this *samadhi*. When we can practice all three together, as we move from *dharana*, through *dyana* into *samadhi*, this process is called *samyama*. In this process, according to Patanjali, the mind becomes very powerful and gains extraordinary psychic abilities, called *siddhis*. Although Patanjali's *Yoga Sutras* go on to describe the *siddhis* in detail, and present a fourth chapter—*kaivalya pada*, we will stop here and sum up what we have learned so far.

Patanjali's *Yoga Sutras* offer an ultimate guidebook for consciousness development. They describe the steps we must take to work with our attitudes and body, and finally, with our mind. Everyone may practice and attain the consciousness expansion, providing they follow the road map described in Chapters 1, 2, and 3 of Patanjali's *Yoga Sutras*. That advanced quality of experience is known as the "super mind" and is the product of trained concentration by managing the mind. As my friend, psychotherapist and accomplished yogi Stephen (Stoma) Parker writes in his recent book *Clearing the Path*:[6] "The secret in the practice of yoga is not so much in following the set of rules, but in gradually, through awareness, improving the attunement…to spiritual Self." As a result, the veil of ignorance is lifted from the mind, which begins to see the reality as is, free of *kleshas* and any conditioning. Such a "clear mind" becomes our instrument to connect with our

---

6   Parker, S. (2017) *Clearing the Path: The Yoga Way to a Clear & Pleasant Mind: Patanjali, Neuroscience and Emotion*. Minnesota, MN: Ahymsa Publishers, pp.107, 227.

own Self and with Universal Divinity/Consciousness. I believe a such a clear mind is what Dr. Miller called "awakened awareness," with all its benefits of extraordinary perception of reality. It knows how to resolve inner conflict, how to decondition the mind from its conditioning and lift it from habitual patterns.

I have presented Patanjali's *Yoga Sutras* in a nutshell as it relates to the subject of spirituality. I strongly encourage everyone to read the translations, of which one of the best (in my opinion) is *Yoga Philosophy of Patanjali with Bhasvati* by Swami Hariharananda Aranya.[7] However, if you read any other classical yogic text—such as *Bhagavad Gita* or *Yoga Vasishta*—they are all guidebooks for spiritual awakening according to the teachings of the Vedanta. From a yoga therapy point of view, however, perhaps equally important to Patanjali's *Yoga Sutras* is a later work, compiled in the 15th century by Svatmarama, titled *Hathapradipika*.

HATHAPRADIPIKA

In the classical texts that teach yoga, the word "yoga" may designate either a practice, or a body of practices, on the one hand, or the goal of such practices, on the other. In Patanjali's *Yoga Sutras* we were introduced to the detailed description of the goal of yoga and to general teaching on how to achieve such a goal. *Hathapradipika*, the best known and most influential text on *Hatha Yoga*, is much more concerned with the body of practices and their health outcomes. For yoga therapists, such a book is a treasure, which should be studied carefully because it describes in detail yogic practices and also lists their health benefits.

Hatha Yoga is supposed to have been taught first by Lord Shiva (the Hindu god of destruction and change) to his consort Parvati. Verse I:10 says: "Hatha yoga is a monastery for those who are afflicted by suffering; for those who practice all kinds of yoga Hatha is the base support." The text compiled by Svatmarama consists of 409 verses, in four chapters, and was also called by other translators *Hathayopgapradipika*.[8]

Ha means sun, *tha* means moon. Yoga is the state of union of these two. The goal of these practices is the purification of *nadis* (subtle energy channels), so that *kundalini* (Divine) energy, inactive at the base of the spine, can be awakened and brought up to the top of the head, through the central channel along the

---

7 Swami Hariharananda Aranya (2012) *Yoga Philosophy of Patanjali with Bhasvati*. Calcutta: University of Calcutta.
8 Swami Digambarji and Raghunathashastri, Pr. (Eds) (1970) *Haṭhapradipika of Svatmarama*. Lonavla, Poona: Maharashtra Kaivalyadhama. There are many versions of the *Hathapradipika*, some listing five chapters and fewer verses.

spine—*sushumna*. Thus *ha* (represented by *pingala nadi*) will meet *tha* (represented by *ida nadi*) at the top of the head. When *kundalini* reaches the top of the head, human conditioning and *karma* is inactive (in Patanjali's *Yoga Sutras* the *kleshas* are burnt) and the yogi experiences bliss and enjoys Superior Consciousness (IV:110), *samadhi*. As we advance in our practices, every step marks the introduction of more and more of the mental and spiritual aspects of yoga. In other words, through the bodily practices of *Hatha Yoga* we will achieve spiritual *Raja Yoga*.

Hathapradipika, as opposed to Patanjali's *Yoga Sutras*, which is regarded as a spiritual yoga (*Raja Yoga*), describes detailed, specific practices, with instructions on how to perform them and what can be expected as a result in terms of health. These instructions are contained in four chapters, and each chapter prepares the *sadhaka* (someone who is dedicated to the path of self-discovery and self-realization) for the practices in the next one:

- Bodily postures: *asana*
- Breathing techniques: *pranayama*
- Gesture or symbolic poses: *mudras*
- Bliss: *samadhi*.

Although *Hathapradipika* does not have a separate chapter for *yamas* and *niyamas*, like Patanjali's *Yoga Sutras*, it does, however, list the qualities to be avoided and those to be practiced in order to achieve the goal of yoga. These are very much applicable in today's world.[9]

The qualities to be avoided are:

- Overeating—which can lead to feeling sluggish mentally and physically, not mentioning any weight gain
- Overexertion—the pace of today's average life can be exhausting, out of balance, and causing high stress, possibly leading to chronic diseases
- Excessive talking—this doesn't leave time for listening, for reflection, for reconnection with oneself
- Adhering to rules too much—although we have rules to make our social life predictable, they should never lead us to not thinking with our own mind
- Excessive public contact—we need some time alone to regain balance in life

---

9   Paraphrased from Jaypalan, L. (2017) "Exploring Sadhaka & Badhaka Tattva." Laura Jay Yoga Blog, November 22. https://laurajayyoga.wordpress.com/2017/11/22/exploring-sadhaka-badhaka-tattva

- Fickle mind—it is difficult to achieve any goals with a mind that is constantly distracted.

On the other hand, here are the qualities that should be promoted if we want to be successful in yoga:

- Enthusiasm— allows to achieve a goal without getting discouraged
- Courage—needed because the ebb and flow of life can be challenging and requires persistence
- Determination—needed because obstacles on the path can be difficult to overcome
- Patience—needed to stay on the path despite challenges
- Resoluteness—confidence and faith in ourselves is a necessary attribute.

Chapter I, *Asana*

In Chapter I, Svatmarama introduces *asanas*. It is worth mentioning that the *asana* went through a metamorphosis from its early classical stages—from being a simple way of sitting for meditation or mantra repetition and breath control to one of the most important diverse and well-documented bodily practices. Svatmarama describes 15 *asanas*, of which seven are sitting postures and eight are not seated and are described for the first time in written form. It is made very clear that an *asana* is a prerequisite for meditation and breath control. In texts that were composed later (16th–18th century), the number of described *asanas* grew to 84, and their therapeutic benefits came to the fore but they were always associated with control of the mind as the end goal. The difference between traditional and modern *asana* practice is worth mentioning.[10]

For traditional yogis it is usually enough to adopt a single position and hold it for a long period of time rather than practice several different *asanas* in succession. The purpose of practicing *asanas* is steadiness, firmness, and nimbleness of the body and in general, good health and lightness of the limbs. *Hathapradipika*, as a first *Hatha Yoga* text, lists the specific benefits of each individual *asana*. *Mayurasana* (peacock pose), for example, is said to get rid of all afflictions of the stomach and spleen and overcome imbalances of the humors. It also destroys tumors. If we have eaten a lot of bad food, it burns it all away and stokes up the digestive fire so that the poison can be digested.

Matsyendra stokes the digestive fire and is a weapon that will destroy a whole

---

10 Mallison, J. and Singleton, M. (2017) *The Roots of Yoga*. London: Penguin Random House.

array of diseases. Through its practice *kundalini* is awakened and a man's semen becomes steady. *Shavasana* (corpse pose) takes away fatigue and relaxes the mind. Svatmarama also introduces the concept of managing the subtle energy within the body. He mentions the use of energy locks (*bandhas*) with *asanas* as well as introducing *prana* and *apana vayus*. Perhaps more important is the concept of *nadis* as a subtle energy channel, which need to be purified by yogic practices. So for yoga therapists, *Hathapradipika* presents a fountain of wisdom with regards to *asanas* as a healing tool.

After describing *asanas* and their health benefits, Svatmarama introduces the concept of yogic diet—*mitahara* (I:58–66). Food is not eaten for our satisfaction, he states, and the stomach should be left a quarter empty. First, the food should be offered to the Almighty. The following types of food are bad for the *Hatha* yogi: bitter, sour, pungent, salty or hot, green vegetables, oil, mustard, alcohol, fish, meat, buttermilk, berries, and garlic. Reheated food with an excess of vegetables is unwholesome and should be avoided. For advanced yogis, wheat, rice, barley, milk, ghee, sugar, butter, honey, dry ginger, cucumber, five leafy vegetables, and rainwater are considered to be wholesome food. Yogis should eat food that is nutritious, sweet, and unctuous, products from cows' milk and nourishing food of their own choice suitable for practicing yoga.

Svatmarama promises further that an individual who untiringly practices yoga in all aspects attains success whether they are young, old, decrepit, diseased, or weak. However, he adds, success is attained by those who practice. How can we attain success without practice? Success in yoga is not achieved by merely reading authentic books. Also, wearing a particular type of dress does not bring success, and nor does talking about yoga. Practicing alone brings success! The practice of *asanas*, *pranayama*, and *mudras* will bring the fruits of yoga—*Raja Yoga*, *samadhi*.

Chapter II, *Pranayama*

Svatmarama presents six preliminary cleansing techniques (*shatkarmas*, II.5.1), as a preparatory practice, which aim at removing gross impurities from the body and render the *sadhaka* fit for more advanced *pranayama* exercises. The term *shatkarma* is older than *Hathapradipika* and may refer to tantric rituals to control other people and for curing diseases. The cleansing process used natural means—water, air, a particular movement of muscles, or using some kind of device. It aims to cleanse such impurities as fat and mucus, or cure a variety of related diseases from the following parts of the body:

- Eyes, nose, throat, and sinuses

- Esophagus and stomach
- Intestines, rectum, and anus.

These *shatkarmas* were:

- *Trataka*, staring at the point without blinking
- *Kapalabhati*, cleansing breathing technique (sometimes also classified as *pranayama*)
- *Neti*, cleansing the nose
- *Dhauti*, cleansing the upper part of the digestive system
- *Nauli*, massage of the stomach by movement of the muscles
- *Basti*, cleansing the lower part of the digestive system.

Those who have an excess of phlegm must practice the six purifying processes (*shatkarmas*) before doing *pranayama*. Those who have *vata*, *pitta*, and *kapha* in a state of equilibrium need not practice them (II:21).

Today, the physical practice of yoga is popularly identified with bodily postures, but in pre-modern India it was breath control that was the defining practice of physical yoga. The ancient yogis were fully aware that behind the overt activity of yogic practice, there was more important covert activity within the living being. So, while referring to overt breathing activity, they always had in their mind a corresponding covert life activity as well. Their idea was that the slower and deeper the respiration, the slower the process of exhaustion and decay of the body. Therefore, they thought of prolonging life by regulating, slowing down, and suspending the breath.[11]

Prana as a life-breath is mentioned from the beginning of India's literary record. *Arthavaveda* states that sublimation of the breath leads to mystical ends, and *pranayama* has remained a key element of yoga practices since the earliest descriptions. The main purpose of *pranayama*, therefore, was to manage *prana* (life force) through the control of the breath and to cleanse impurities from the subtle energy channels—*nadis*. *Sushumna* is the *nadi* that runs along the spinal cord up to the top of the brain. Yogis often speak of *prana* ascending to the top of the brain, along *sushumna nadi*. Cleansing this *nadi* and pulling the *prana* along this *nadi* is preparation to awakening and raising *kundalini*. Svatmarama describes different *pranayama* techniques using *surya* or *pingala nadi* (right nostril), and *chandra*

---

[11] Swami Digambarji and Raghunathashastri, Pr. (Eds) (1970) *Haṭhapradipika of Svatmarama*. Lonavla, Poona: Maharashtra Kaivalyadhama.

or *ida nadi* (left nostril). The first is known to be stimulating and the latter to being relaxing. The practice of *pranayama* arouses *kundalini*, which raises through *sushumna* to the top of the head, and the success of *Hatha Yoga* is achieved (II:6).

Pranayama as a therapeutic tool is extremely potent, and if practiced properly can eliminate all diseases (II:16). However, improper practice of *pranayama* gives rise to all sorts of diseases, such as hiccups, asthma, a cough, disturbed sleep, headache, or pain in the ear or eyes are due to mismanagement of *prana* (II:17). Therefore, breath control should be developed gradually with the help of a teacher, otherwise it may harm the practitioner. With proper practice, however, gastric heat is increased, and good health is secured (II:20). *Pranayama* should be practiced four times in 24 hours, so every four hours.

As long as the breath is controlled in the body, the mind is calm (II:40). This is predicated on the notion that the mind and breath are inextricably linked. This connection, which is first taught in the *Chandogya Upanishad*, appears to underpin the teaching of both Patanjali's *Yoga Sutras* and *Hathapradipika*. Controlling the mind by controlling the breath is said to lead directly to liberation. What a fantastic pearl of teaching for yoga therapists!

When all the subtle energy channels—*nadis*—have been purified by correctly managing breathing, the *prana* enters *sushumna* and the mind becomes perfectly steady. Such steadiness of the mind is a supramental state and may lead to attaining supranatural powers (*siddhis*) (II:41–43).

Verses II:39–46 detail eight different *pranayama* techniques with the addition of locks—*mula bandha* (root lock) and *jalandhara bandha* (chin lock). The eight *pranayamas* described in detail are: *surya bhedana, ujjayi, sitkari, sitali, bhastrika, bhramari, murcha,* and *plavini*. For us, however, as yoga therapists, most important are the health benefits mentioned for each one of the techniques:

- *Surya bhedana* (*surya* = sun, *bhedan* = activate). Benefits: May improve circulation, rejuvenate cells, purify blood and remove parasites, balance *vata* disorders, and calm *pitta*. Helpful for tremors in the feet, neuropathy of the feet, tightening feeling of the feet, sciatica cramps, rigidity of the knee, stiffness of joints and shoulder muscles, and puffiness of the body and fingers. Also for the emotionally reserved, irritability, excessive talking, insomnia, and fickleness of the mind and intellect.

- *Ujjayi* (to raise, also called victorious breath). Benefits: May remove throat diseases and increase temperature of the body. Helpful in low blood pressure, dropsy, assimilation problems, increasing stamina and agility, and removing nerve disorders like stress and depression. Helpful in balancing *kapha*.

- *Sitkari* (hissing breath). Benefits: May bring luster, especially on the face, conquer thirst and if excess, normalize it; the yogi may gain control over one's body.

- *Sitali* (cooling breath). Benefits: May heal spleen disorder, prevent formation of tumors, remove *pitta* disorders by balancing it, helpful for high blood pressure, removing heat from the body, useful in fever, normalizing hunger and thirst. Sitali brings down *pitta* by addressing the root of imbalance.

- *Bhastrika* (bellows breath). Benefits: May cure the diseases of *vata*, *pitta*, and *kapha* and increase gastric heat. Helpful in balancing all *doshas*, increases body temperature, useful in low blood pressure, may infuse vigor and stamina, alertness and memory, and remove depression. Awakens *kundalini*, pierces the three *granthis*—*Brahma*, *Vishnu*, and *Rudra* (energy knots at the navel, heart, and throat).

- *Bhramari* (bee breath). Benefits: May be beneficial in all cardiovascular dysfunctions including high blood pressure, increases concentration and ability to control the mind. Leads to blissful meditation.

- *Kapalabhati* (skull shining breath). Although mentioned in the *shatkarmas*, *kapalabhati* is often regarded as a *pranayama* technique. Benefits: May rejuvenate the brain cells (*kapha dosha*, *vishosini*), curing the *kapha*.

Chapter III, *Mudras*

Chapter III starts with explaining that all yogic practices aim at awakening *kundalini*, the dormant power in man.[12] When *kundalini* is awakened to action, all the subtle energy centers (*chakras*) and knots (*granthis*, obstruction) are pierced by *prana* and the *nadis* are cleansed. *Kundalini* is then free to travel to the top of the head[13] and

---

12 The yogis believe that this power in the form of a serpent sleeps at the base of the spine obstructing the entrance to *sushumna*, the main *nadi* along the spine of the human. Her slumber binds the ignorant to the worldliness.

13 The yogis believe that through practices the Supreme Realization is attained when the sleeping *Kundalini* awakens, and rising up the *sushumna* reaches *brahmarandhra*, the highest center in the brain, which they call the spotless abode of Brahman, the one Supreme Reality.

the mind becomes objectless, achieving the highest mental state. *Mudras* are the next step in difficulty to practice awakening *kundalini*.

Although *Hathapradipika* is dated to the 15th century, there are references to ascetics practicing similar techniques from the time of Buddha onwards.

Svatmarama continues to list 10 *mudras* with a detailed description of how to perform them and a list of the benefits of each: *mahamudra, mahabandha, mahavedha, khechari mudra, uddiyana bandha, mula bandha, jalandhara bandha, virpitikarni, vajroli,* and *shakti chalana mudra* (III:1–6). We are particularly interested in the health benefits these mudras may present to a practitioner:

- *Mahamudra.* May heal diseases such as consumption, skin disease, constipation, glandular enlargement, indigestion, and many others (III:7–17).
- *Mahabandha.* May bestow great *siddhis* (extraordinary powers) upon the *sadhaka* (III:18–23).
- *Mahavedha.* May prevent wrinkles, gray hair, and bodily tremors (III:24–29).

These three *mudras* may delay old age and death, increase gastric heat, and bring supernatural powers.

- *Khechari mudra.* Someone who has mastered this *mudra* is free from disease, fatigue, death, sleep, hunger, thirst, or stupor. They are not bound by *karma* (the fruit of their action), and nor are they the subject of the cycle of death and birth. Mastering this *mudra* results in Self-realization, the highest state of consciousness (III:31–53).

- *Uddiyana bandha* (upward abdominal lock). This is the most effective of all *bandhas*; the old person practicing *uddiyana* becomes young (III:54–59).

- *Mula bandha* (root lock). Causes downward subtle energy (*apanavayu*) to rise and meet upward subtle energy (*prana*), thus entering *sushumna*, awakening *kundalini* to travel up to unite with Bindu at the top of the head. As a result the old become young, and urine and ordure diminish (III:60–68).

- *Jalandhara bandha* (chin lock). Regulates *vata*, one of the three *doshas*.

- *Viparita karani* (inverted pose). Should be learned not from books but from someone who has mastered the pose. Wrinkles and gray hair disappear.

Svatmarama finishes Chapter III with the promise—"By an untiring practice of *asanas*, *pranayama* and *mudras* the *sushumna* becomes easy for *kundalini* to travel" (III:120). All the practices should be done with a concentrated mind—the yogis should never allow the mind to wander during the practice (III:123).

Chapter IV, *Samadhi*

This chapter is dedicated to *samadhi*, presented by Svatmarama as a state of equilibrium, which creates union between *Jivatma* (our individual Self) with *Paramatma* (Divine, or Universal Consciousness) (IV:6, 7). Once again, the interdependence of mental activity and respiration is stressed—when one is active, the other is active too. Therefore, the restraint of respiration leads to the restraint of mental activities of the individual, allowing for union (IV:21–25).

So far, we have considered two of perhaps the most popular yogic texts that were translated directly from source in Sanskrit and published with commentaries by many revered yogic masters. These two are representative of the yogic classical opus because they share the same elements—yoga as a goal and yogic practices as the path to reach that goal. And what is the goal of yoga? Contrary to the common belief in the West, the goal of yoga is not having a nice figure or being flexible or generally feeling better. The goal of yoga is *samadhi*—the state of expanded consciousness that produces the highest state of mind possible for a human being.

All different paths of yoga—*Bhakti*, *Raja*, *Jnana*, *Karma*, or *Tantra*—lead in the same direction, to achieve the state of beingness in union with Divine/Universal Consciousness. Marion called it the ninth and final stage of human spiritual development—*the nondual consciousness of identity with God*.[14] Rohr also describes this as the ninth stage of spiritual development: *We are now fully detached from our own self-image and living in God's image of us—which includes and loves both the good and the bad. We experience true serenity and freedom. This is the peace the world cannot give (see John 14:27) and full resting in God.*[15] Myss called it living in the penthouse. The highest state of mind possible for human beings has infinite awareness, understanding, and insight.

Translating these statements to our everyday vocabulary, the goal of yoga is transcending our limitations and conditioning, and through self-mastery moving towards Self-realization or Enlightenment. Perhaps not everyone is able to achieve the highest state of mind possible to human beings. However, everyone is on the

---

14 Marion, J. (2004) *The Death of the Mythic God: The Rise of Evolutionary Spirituality*. Charlottesville, VA: Hampton Roads Publishing Company, Inc.
15 Rohr, R. (2024) "A maturing spirituality." Daily Meditations, Center for Action and Contemplation, June 17. https://cac.org/daily-meditations/a-maturing-spirituality

path to expand their level of consciousness as they grow up and mature, whether they know it or not. The key concept here, though, is that yoga as a path becomes a journey of self-discovery, offering individuals the tools to unlock their full potential and lead fulfilling and happy lives.

These comprehensive systems include a code of ethical conduct—*yamas* and *niyamas* as the first steps of yoga in *Patanjali's Yoga Sutras*. In *Hathapradipika*, the qualities to be avoided (don'ts) or promoted (dos) are not listed as explicitly as in Patanjali's *Yoga Sutras*, but are mentioned in many verses. *Hathapradipika* also touches on the diet that is helpful in achieving yogic goals. Both recommend *asanas*, with *Hathapradipika* describing the postures and listing the health benefits of *asanas* and *pranayama*.[16] Both recommend *pranayama* (breathing techniques), stressing their importance over all other practices. There is also an interesting difference in emphasis in the two texts re: pranayama. Patanjali focuses on making the breath long and subtle until kevala kumbhaka spontaneously appears. HYP is much more about conscious manipulation of the breath and prana and conscious and intentional suspension of breath. Patanjali's *Yoga Sutras*, also called *Raja Yoga*, specifically devotes a whole chapter to working and training the mind. Finally, both texts point to a deeper, spiritual dimension of yoga, as a way of healing and release from suffering. This is a complete system for personal growth and well-being.

In summary, we presented a short review of two classical yoga texts as they relate to yoga therapy and spirituality. Patanjali's *Yoga Sutras* and *Hathapradipika* present yoga as a profound and comprehensive system, addressing the complexities of human suffering and promoting holistic well-being across physical, mental, environmental, and spiritual dimensions. These two texts, and many other classical yogic texts, recommend the road map outlining the path a person (*sadhaka*) must take, practices a person must master to come closer to self-realization. Perhaps the quintessence of spirituality in yogic texts is contained in Patanjali's first *sutra* in Chapter II, the ability to surrender to Divine will and let go of the end goal (*Ishvara pranidhana*).

---

16 The research on *pranayama* confirms some claims; however, no research yet exists on a single *asana* or *mudra* to confirm the claims listed in the *Hathapradipika*. Also, some descriptions of benefits are expressed in poetic language and may contain exaggerated statements.

CHAPTER 6

Yoga Therapy as a Spiritual Path

Wrong knowledge (ignorance of reality) is the main problem in life.
PATANJALI'S *YOGA SUTRAS*, 2:5 (WRITTEN IN THE EARLY CENTURIES BC)

Yoga focuses on how to achieve balance for all levels of the body—physical, energetic, emotional, mental, and spiritual. As we saw in Chapter 5, at the heart of all yogic classical texts is bringing balance to human life and the expansion of consciousness through various practices.

We may also think of the four aspects of human existence at the level of:

- body
- mind
- energy (*prana*)
- consciousness (spirit).

Likewise, we can think of yoga therapy as comprised of several aspects:

- It is a preventive discipline, dealing mostly with the physical body, and includes practices, yogic diet (*mitahara*), and the ability to keep the body in a relaxed state.

- It is healing science, providing the opportunity to restore physical, energetic, emotional, and mental balance based predominantly today on *Tantra Yoga* (*Hathapradipika*). It also includes yogic counselling and supporting the client emotionally.

- It is a transformative tool, which creates an irreversible shift in *prana* and consciousness (spirit), which, in turn, brings balance to the body. This last aspect is the most comprehensive and highest skill in yoga therapy. It moves the client from lack of self-awareness to a state of dispassionate witnessing of their inner and outer states. It also brings the client to understanding who they really are—to disidentify with their body or thoughts and to reconnecting with their higher Self (or Divinity within). Such a transformation of consciousness is the answer to solving all the problems humanity is facing today. And it is yoga therapy at its highest level.

Knowledge of the physical body and its functionality is easily available through medical science. To a certain degree the same applies to the brain and nervous system, although Western science is still struggling with the concept of the mind. But psychiatry and Western psychology knowledge is widely available.

Perhaps this is why the majority of yoga therapists focus their work primarily on the client's body and, to a certain degree, on their mind, but with the omission of *prana* and consciousness (spirituality). In other words, many yoga professionals use yoga therapy as a healing science and not as a tool to transform the whole human being.

Why is this, you may ask? The answer, I believe, lies in the fact that knowledge of spirituality, consciousness, and/or *prana*, unlike the body and brain, is not readily available and easily accessible in books supplied by other disciplines. We must dive deep into yogic philosophy and yogic texts—not an easy task for the Westerner—to slowly gain some understanding. Even so, all that information may not be easily accepted by the Western mind, as neither consciousness nor *prana* can yet be measured by Western science.

We may find texts describing consciousness, spirituality, or *prana*, but none of this will be properly understood unless we experience these ourselves. This is where intellectual knowledge must be augmented by personal experience, because without experience, we are unable to properly apply that knowledge.

This is why the spiritual journey must be the goal of every yoga professional. Only when we "clear" our own vision through *sadhana* are we are able to perceive our client as a whole, without any distortions and projections. Perhaps our professional responsibility therefore is to work on transforming our own level of consciousness first, possibly moving from one state of consciousness to a higher one, so that we can be of better service to our clients. *In my opinion, this process should be listed in the core competencies of every serious yoga therapy training course. Daily yoga sadhana should be required from every yoga therapist as long as they practice this profession.* We will describe later how we see this process as a healing taking place in our clients.

Before we go any further, we should understand the difference between transformation and change. When I have a toothache and take a painkiller, the toothache goes away—my level of pain changes. When the painkiller stops working, the level of pain comes back to its previous state. Think of change as a pendulum, swinging back and forth. When you take a painkiller for toothache, the pain subsides temporarily, only to return when the medication wears off. That's mere change—a temporary shift in state.

The journey of transformation is far more profound than simple change. Imagine a symphony where every note represents a different aspect of our being—physical, energetic, emotional, mental, and spiritual. Each one plays its unique part in the grand orchestration of human existence.

Once you transform your consciousness, you do not go back to the previous state. It's like a butterfly emerging from its chrysalis—there's no going back. When you truly transform, you ascend to a new level of understanding, much like climbing to a higher floor in a building, to use Caroline Myss's metaphor from earlier. Your perspective broadens, your values deepen, and your entire worldview shifts permanently. Your understanding of life changes and your motivations change. You understand the lower level of consciousness you had, but now you live from a higher level. (All the stories in Part 2 of this book are testimonies to such transformations brought about by yoga practices.)

What makes yoga unique in the landscape of healing practices is its comprehensive approach to transformation. It doesn't just work with the body or mind in isolation. Instead, it provides a framework for addressing the root causes of imbalance, touching the deepest aspects of our being. The key to unlocking this potential lies not in mere intellectual understanding, but in personal experience. Like learning to swim, no amount of theoretical knowledge can replace the actual experience of being in the water.

The spiritual aspects of yoga, the possibility of the transformation of consciousness and knowledge, and the management of *prana* differentiates yoga therapy from all other complementary disciplines in healthcare. More importantly it provides the framework to influence the deepest aspects of diseases and ability to restore the innermost imbalances. It is yoga therapy at its highest and most potent level. But to be able to use the deeper aspects of yoga therapy to guide our clients, we must first experience these transformations ourselves. To truly harness the transformative power of yoga therapy, we must first walk the path ourselves. Only by experiencing the reorganization of our own *prana* and the expansion of our own consciousness can we authentically assist others on this profound journey of healing and self-discovery. To make this point explicit, what follows are my experiences at the beginning of my yoga journey, when I met my teacher.

At one of my lectures in Canada, I met someone who everyone was calling "guru." After a short conversation he invited me to his ashram for a few weeks. I had no knowledge of yoga, an ashram or a "guru," but I was at the stage of my life when I was open to an adventure, and so I went for three weeks. Weeks extended to months, and in the end I spent over three years living in the ashram as a staff member. I found it to be a battle ground for my ego. I soon learned that the ashram environment offers a metaphoric express highway to spiritual development, under the watchful eye of the guru/teacher. Relationships between staff members were constantly challenging, and pushing each one of us to see our own conditioning and unresolved issues. This was often a very painful process, and by any means not for the faint-hearted.

My teacher—Sri Vasudeva—was very approachable, yet often, instead of offering consolation or explanation, I was met with additional challenge. Somehow, he always saw right through me, and instead of answering my question he would address the issues that lay behind my question. I would often leave the conversation confused, and had to spend some time digesting what had been said. He had a way of beating my ego to a pulp with no mercy, although he would do so in the most loving way.

There was much more to my stay in the ashram. Here are my notes of the training I was lucky to receive:

> At the beginning I didn't consider Sri Vasudeva as someone special despite the reverence other people showed him. To me he was nice, perhaps a highly developed human being working towards the benefit of others. However, I noticed that often my mind would become empty in his presence. My responsibilities required a lot of interactions with him and almost daily I needed to ask for his decisions in many matters. However, when we met, quite often I found that all the questions were gone, and I had a completely empty mind. That was quite embarrassing...
>
> One day I asked him: "How is it that when I am in your presence all my questions vanish and I cannot even remember them?"
>
> He smiled and said: "In every human interaction there is an exchange of subtle energy. Like between a magnet and metal shavings. The magnet has much more centered, therefore stronger energy and influences metal shavings along its energy lines. The same with us—my energy influences you in a particular way and all your intellect activities change. In the future simply write the questions down on a piece of paper before you come to me."

That was something very new to me—my first aware experience with subtle energy.

The next experience was even stranger. I must mention here that before I entered the ashram, I was already a self-taught meditator of 15 years. I never had a meditation teacher per se, and my meditation was never formally evaluated. I simply liked it and practiced it without any guidance, not realizing that this is yoga. In consequence my meditation was raw, intuitive, and unguided.

One day my teacher wanted to evaluate my meditation skills. We sat in his office and meditated silently together. I went really deep. I was aware of the environment, but at the same time I entered a state of perfect pose—physically, mentally, and psychologically. Physically—I was in perfect equilibrium sitting comfortably on my cushion. Mentally and psychologically– my mind was still, and I was sitting in inner silence. I do not know how long we sat there but it felt like a very short moment, when he started to guide me in our meditation. I really didn't want to come out! I forced myself to open my eyes, but it took me another few minutes before I was able to move my body.

However, soon after I left his office, I realized that I felt very strange. It almost felt like I was energetically dissected, and all the parts of me were totally misaligned. That sensation was very difficult to describe—I was disorientated, but not in a bad way, there was a feeling of being suspended somewhere in the air, and at the same time the parts of my body felt strangely out of synch in their movement. All the impressions and sounds seemed to be amplified and intolerable, as if I couldn't process them.

I went to my room and sat on a chair facing the white wall. That felt good. No input from the environment, peace and quiet around—I sat there for few hours and didn't want to move. It felt as if all the fragments that were part of me were out of synch and needed downtime to come back into harmony and synchronize. This was my first Wall Time.

In more than three years in the ashram, I had many such Wall Times. It would happen after some prolonged interaction with the teacher, or after usual chanting or meditation sessions in the community hall. I never knew when it would happen, but I sure knew when it did!

Sometimes it took few hours of Wall Time to come back to inner balance. But sometimes it took days… I guess something was working for me and on me. My ego was certainly not in charge of the process. Perhaps all the yogic practices in the ashram schedule, plus the community and the strong presence of well-organized energy, were clearing up my innermost being.

About a year-and-a-half into my stay at the ashram I started to feel held by some kind of energy. It was a very physical sensation, as if there was someone literally wrapping their arms around me and holding me in safety. I feel it sometimes to this day—protected, held, and guided...

At the end of my third year in the ashram something shifted. Suddenly Vasudeva's usual very friendly demeanor changed, and our every occasional interchange became rather unpleasant for me. When meeting him on the ashram grounds, occasionally he would say something vile to me, such as: "Namaskar Lee... Tell me, who did you have a fight with today?"

This went on for several weeks. At the beginning I reacted with anger, although I didn't let myself be provoked into a conversation. I didn't understand why he had turned on me this way, what had changed, and why I deserved such treatment. After all, I contributed so much to the ashram! I was busy creating CDs and DVDs with his meditations, I was documenting his work on videotapes creating archives, I was accompanying him on the keyboard twice a day at the community chants. What the hell was wrong with him?!

I was considering leaving the ashram, but I was working on a major project and thought I should finish before I left. I started avoiding any direct contact with him. My anger subsided and I simply didn't care anymore how he treated me. Somehow internally I knew that my work here made sense, and I focused on finishing the projects. If I saw him coming down to the building where my office was, I would close the door. One day, about two months into this treatment, as I was coming out of my office, I saw Vasudeva standing at the entrance to the building. We stood there for a moment, looking at each other. I was waiting for him to say something nasty, as usual. Instead, he said quietly: "Are you going to leave me? Everything I did was with love in my heart for you."

I understood immediately—his job as a spiritual teacher was to lead me to find my "inner guru" within myself and to stop depending on him. A month later I was diagnosed with cancer, and I had to come back to Canada for treatment. By then the connection to my Self, my inner guru, was open, though.

THE SACRED DANCE: TRADITIONAL YOGA TRAINING VS. MODERN ADAPTATIONS

Perhaps such trainings can happen only in the ashram's high-energy environment, which includes daily yoga discipline (*sadhana*), selfless service (*seva*), and a teacher–student (*guru–shishya*) long-term relationship. All this is in line with the Indian classical tradition, which understood that the way to connect with inner Self/Divinity is through beating the ego into submission.

The contrast between traditional ashram-based training and contemporary Western approaches reveals not just methodological differences but also fundamental philosophical divergences that shape the very essence of yogic experience. In the traditional ashram setting, transformation isn't just a possibility; it's inevitable. The environment operates like a spiritual pressure cooker, where three essential elements create an alchemical process:

- *Daily sadhana:* The rigorous discipline of daily practices creates a rhythm that gradually dissolves the ego's resistance. Each sunrise meditation, every *pranayama* session becomes a thread in the fabric of transformation.

- *Seva:* Through selfless service, students learn to act without attachment to results. Washing dishes, sweeping floors—these mundane tasks become profound spiritual practices when approached with devotional awareness.

- *Guru–shishya relationship:* This ancient mentorship model provides a mirror for self-reflection and a channel for transmission of the subtle energies that catalyze inner awakening.

The shift to online yoga training, while democratizing access, has created what I call a "spiritual bandwidth problem." Just as a video call can't fully capture the nuances of in-person communication, digital yoga instruction struggles to transmit the subtle energetic exchanges that traditionally facilitate deeper transformation.

Here lies another of our modern dilemmas: We seek spiritual growth while simultaneously clinging to ego-affirming individualism. We insist on being sensitive to our client's feelings. It's like trying to empty and fill a cup at the same time. In addition, the Western approach often treats yoga as a commodity—another self-improvement tool in our wellness toolkit—rather than a very disciplined path of self-transcendence and transformation. However, I don't believe all is lost. Perhaps the solution lies not in completely abandoning modern approaches, but in creating hybrid models that honor both tradition and contemporary reality. Consider:

- Establishing long-term mentorship programs that combine in-person intensives with online support
- Integrating *seva* projects into local communities
- Developing new frameworks for ego transcendence that speak to the Western psyche without compromising the essential teaching.

For the next generation of yoga professionals, the challenge will be to bridge these worlds. While it's true that many may miss the depth of traditional training, there is also an opportunity to pioneer new approaches that maintain spiritual integrity while meeting modern practitioners where they are.

The key lies in understanding that while the methods may evolve, the essential truth remains: the journey beyond ego to Self-realization requires dedication, guidance, and a willingness to be transformed. This exploration reveals not just the challenges facing modern yoga education, but also the broader question of how ancient wisdom can be authentically transmitted in our digital age. The answer may lie not in lamenting what's lost, but in creatively reimagining what's possible.

SADHANA AS A CORE COMPETENCY

Offering the possibility of self-discovery leading to a fulfilling, healthier, and happier life for the client is the primary calling for the yoga therapist. However, to be able to offer that the yoga therapist has to first experience and continue walking the path themselves. That is why both texts (Patanjali's *Yoga Sutras* and *Hathapradipika*) explicitly stress experiential learning through daily yogic practices—*sadhana*.

We may read about yoga, yet without personal daily practice we may never learn the deeper meaning of these practices and their hidden spiritual and health benefits. Each practice, when mastered, does what it was designed to do—increases our state of consciousness. Therefore, we must understand that daily *sadhana* is a core competency for the yoga therapist. These practices lead to expanding our consciousness, thus increasing the yoga therapist's professional competency.

Yoga is a science based not merely on logical reasoning; it was originally taught by seers who experienced the truths through direct realization and personal experiences, later articulated in classical texts. Yoga is therefore known primarily through experiential knowledge. Perhaps the most important feature of yoga is our ability to subdue the flow of thoughts through the mind, which is developed into a habit with consistent practice—*sadhana*. As we gain proficiency in *sadhana*, we develop the purity of the inner instrument of cognition (Patanjali's *Yoga Sutras* 1:47). Such purity of our inner instrument of perception gives us the power to know the things as they are, objectively, with no trace of any personal influence. It retains and sustains the truth alone, with no trace of misconception.

The concept of mind in yoga philosophy is much more far-reaching than in the West. It postulates existence of the mind field, which encompasses both personal and nonpersonal "energy and information"[1] on self and Self. The way to reconnect to this mind field is to become aware and examine the source *of the activity of thought*, the source of the "chatter" in our heads. Such awareness will lift the veil of ignorance, clear the *kleshas*, and reconnect us to the Self, moving us towards the state of yoga.

The promise is simple—for us as yoga therapists, to maintain daily *sadhana* means inching towards the Self (*atman*) by transforming our own consciousness. As yoga therapists we may begin to see inner connections between all things and people. We may begin to sense the subtle flows that take place within our relationship with our client, within any relationship, family, organization, or society. We also may sense intuitively the natural hierarchies of the great chain of being and consciousness. We may start striving to cooperate with that flow and maximize abundance, both material and spiritual, for all beings. The development of such abilities is essential for yoga therapists. And the way to reach these abilities is experiential, through personal daily *sadhana*.

There has been recent research on how yoga impacts spirituality. In 2019, Kwok,[2] with her team, conducted randomized clinical trials for over 130 patients with Parkinson's disease in Hong Kong. They found that eight weeks of 90-minute mindfulness yoga resulted in a reduction in anxiety and depressive symptoms and *an increase in spiritual well-being*. A similar increase in spiritual well-being was reported later by Bryan's[3] team in 2021. The same year an interesting systematic review of the relationship between spirituality and yoga was published in *Frontiers of Psychology* by Csala and colleagues.[4] They studied the available empirical research on spirituality, and found that practicing yoga increased *conscious interactions with others, compassion, trust in Higher Power, and improved spiritual well-being*. Further, they found that yoga practice was positively associated with *spiritual aspirations, search for wisdom, an integrative worldview, a sense of meaning and peace, and happiness within*.

---

1 Siegel, D. (2010) *Mindsight: The New Science of Personal Transformation*. New York: Bantam Books, p.52.
2 Kwok, J. Y. Y., Kwan, J. C. Y., Auyeung, M., Mok, V. C. T., et al. (2019) "Effects of mindfulness yoga vs stretching and resistance training exercises on anxiety and depression for people with Parkinson disease: A randomized clinical trial." *JAMA Neurology* 76, 7, 755–763. doi: 10.1001/jamaneurol.2019.0534.
3 Bryan, S., Zipp, G., and Breitkreuz, D. (2021) "The effects of mindfulness meditation and gentle yoga on spiritual well-being in cancer survivors: A pilot study." *Alternative Therapies in Health and Medicine* 27, 3, 32–38. PMID: 33128538.
4 Csala, B., Springinsfeld, C. M., and Köteles, F. (2021) "The relationship between yoga and spirituality: A systematic review of empirical research." *Frontiers in Psychology* 12, 695939. doi: 10.3389/fpsyg.2021.695939.

The development of higher perceptions (*visayavati*) also brings about tranquility of the mind (Patanjali's *Yoga Sutras* 1:35) in the yoga therapist. Higher sense perception indicates the ability to perceive the subtle features of the object of the senses. Even more importantly, with consistent long-term practice of *sadhana*, the practitioner's mind becomes quiet and able to perceive the true features of the object of contemplation (Patanjali's *Yoga Sutras* 1:41).

Therefore, yoga *sadhana* is not to feel better or for self "maintenance," as many seem to believe. Yoga *sadhana* leads to expansion of consciousness, to the state of yoga. Daily *sadhana* attenuates our own conditioning and *karmic samskaras*, allowing us, yoga therapists, to perceive the true causes of health problems in our clients.

Sadhana makes us better yoga therapists, and thus it belongs to core professional competencies as long as the yoga therapist is professionally active. Just like a blind man cannot give instructions regarding anything concerning the visual properties of the object, so the teaching of the person who has not themselves realized any truth through personal experience cannot relate to any achievable principle. Hence *sadhana* is the basis of all yoga studies.

But what is *sadhana*?

Sadhana, a spiritual yogic practice, is the means by which we attenuate the afflictions (*kleshas*) so that we can reconnect with our own true Self/Divinity. Consistent daily practice and renunciation are the means to our happiness and well-being (Patanjali's *Yoga Sutras* 1:12). Moreover, we will only benefit if we maintain consistent practice. Concentration with strong mental, moral, and physical discipline is the aim of *sadhana*. *No matter which yogic practice we include in sadhana, concentration and awareness must be part of it, otherwise it is not yoga*. That practice must be continued for a long time, daily, without a break, and with unwavering devotion (Patanjali's *Yoga Sutras* 1:14). After some time, such practice becomes a way of life and awareness seeps into every awaken moment. Such yogic *sadhana* becomes the means of removing impurities from the person and leads to attainment of discrimination. A key consequence of yogic *sadhana* is to bring to the surface skills that are inherent in everyone.

YOGA PROFESSIONAL, KNOW THYSELF!

Yogic classical texts explicitly mention that the knowledge of Self, attained through concentration of the mind, is the highest virtue. Happiness is the result of virtue—knowledge of Self or the state of liberation brings about peace and the highest form of welfare. This correlates with Marion's concept of human evolution as the evolution of our consciousness. As we do our daily *sadhana*, we may move to a higher level of consciousness, of beginning contemplatives—level 6 on Marion's scale. Psychic state is the state of expanded, awakened awareness, where we perceive information by more than just our five senses—super-sensuous awareness.

The super-sensuous knowledge, vast or little, that is found in any being is the seed of omniscience. That seed has grades of development in each human and is thus capable of increasing continuously with proper practice (Patanjali's *Yoga Sutras* 2:25). Our ability, as yoga therapists, to develop such extra-sensuous abilities is most valuable in our professional work with clients. Clients are often not aware of the cause of their problem, are often not able to express it with words. Moreover, things that are subtle, hidden from view, cannot be known by ordinary observation.

One researcher into parapsychology—Dean Radin[5]—is very clear in his book *Supernormal: Science, Yoga, and the Evidence for Extraordinary Psychic Abilities*.[6] The connection between the mystical and the miraculous is provided by yoga, a path for *practical mystical development*. That path explicitly includes the development of miraculous phenomena, or, more precisely, of super-marvelous phenomena that appear to be miraculous. Patanjali dedicated the whole third chapter of the *Yoga Sutras* to describing these super-marvelous phenomena called *siddhis*.

The *siddhis* are a refined expression of everyone's potential, Radin continues. But our distracted minds and our beliefs, acting as filters to what we allow ourselves to perceive, prevent us from realizing this potential. Therefore, we need to train our mind to become progressively more sensitive to the holistic nature of reality that we cannot normally apprehend.

THE WAY

To achieve this, Patanjali outlines the path—yoga *sadhana*—which can take us there. Through such yogic training, yogis and yoginis have developed techniques to do things science cannot yet adequately explain. This tells us that the modern understanding of the human mind, which is based on neuroscience, has completely overlooked a fundamental aspect of our capacities and potentials. Both science and religious scholars have prematurely discarded stories about the *siddhis* as mere superstitions. In Part 2 of this book we will have a chance to read about some very unusual, some unexplainable, personal stories of long-term yoga practitioners.

---

5   https://en.wikipedia.org/wiki/Dean_Radin
6   Radin, D. (2013) *Supernormal: Science, Yoga, and the Evidence for Extaordinary Psychic Abilities.* New York: Deepak Chopra Books.

In simple terms, yoga seeks to purify the link between material and consciousness, so that the relationship between our physical world and consciousness becomes clearer. In the process of clarification, the undistracted mind begins to see the true relationships between matter and consciousness. *Siddhis* are the side effect of that insight. When the link is completely clear, enlightenment is said to occur. That's the whole story of yoga in a nutshell.[7]

Robert Butera puts it in simple terms:

> To me the whole field of yoga therapy today is missing the essence of yoga—the spiritual aspect of it. When you help people drop deep into themselves and become more spiritual, that's the magic that the *sadhana* brings about. People will feel the relief of suffering even without removing the disease. The claim of minimizing suffering by showing *asana* seems to me to be ridiculous. I show them *asana* as a bonus, once they realize their True Self, they will do *asana* if only because it's good for the body. Some yoga therapists use *asana* and *pranayama* as a magic to relief the suffering—which is a concept put upside down.

In *Mahabharata* it has been said: "As a man on the hill-top sees the man on the plains, so one having ascended to the palace of knowledge and becoming free from sorrow sees others who are suffering." It seems obvious, then, that the yoga therapist's responsibility is to hone this super-sensuous perception through personal *sadhana*. This allows the yoga therapist to tune in to the client and provide more accurate and deeper assessment of their client. The ability of the yoga therapist to sense what is behind the words, what is unspoken by the client, belongs to the core competency of yoga therapy. The ability to include the super-sensuous information in the assessment of the client marks the excellence of the yoga therapist.

THE PRESENCE

Eckhart Tolle talks about teaching "presence" in interacting and working with others.[8] To do that we need to achieve certain inner qualities. First is the ability to transcend the mental and emotional conditioning of our own mind and become accepting of the present moment. This means the ability to resolve our own burden of past experiences and our burden of anxiety of the future. This, in turn, results in

---

7   Radin, D. (2013) *Supernormal: Science, Yoga, and the Evidence for Extaordinary Psychic Abilities*. New York: Deepak Chopra Books.
8   Tolle, E. (2024) "The world needs you as a teacher of presence." Miniseries [online], October. https://teachings.eckharttolle.com/etn-school-of-awakening-presence-at-work

the ability to live in the now, to honor the now and be grateful for what is, and to live in the arising "presence" within. Such an inner shift brings a quality of deeper stillness of presence as we listen to the client.

This power of presence gained through the tools of yoga therapy opens our intuition to play perhaps an equal or even bigger role than the intellectual knowledge of the subject. We still apply all the tools we have learned, but our ability to hold the presence by being in awakened awareness expands our interaction with our client to a much deeper level. It's important to note that Dr. Miller's achieving awakened awareness corresponds with yoga philosophy (see Chapter 2).

When we are in achieving awareness—*surya* mode—we are in "doing," in well-organized, goal-oriented, rule-abiding action. The energy flow—*prana*—is dominant in *pingala nadi*. When we are in awakened awareness, we operate in *chandra* mode, in the "being," in the flow of creativity moved by something transcendent to us, unrestrained by rules and regulations, without attachment to the end result. In this case *prana* flow is dominant in *ida nadi*. As we evolve and learn to integrate—both achieving and awakened awareness, the "doing" and the "being"—in yogic terms we achieve integration of *pingala* and *ida*.

That integration causes the *prana* to flow through the main *nadi*—*sushumna*—as we are now in the "inaction in action." This is when our sensitivity is refined enough to be able to access subtle energy information. As we open ourselves to the information coming from the inner Self (*atman*), we are able to act on that guidance with integrity. In other words, as we integrate *pingala* and *ida*, we achieve the state of yoga. (The *surya*, *chandra*, and *sushumna nadis* concept comes from the *Upanishads*[9] and is the base of the classical text *Hathayogapradipika*[10].)

ARE WE READY?

It is critical to realize that the yoga therapist's ability to provide spiritual care to their client seems to be somewhat limited to the degree of their own spiritual development as well as the level of their consciousness. As Marion mentions, people at each level of consciousness have their own worldviews. They see and understand the world in a different way from people at other levels. At the same

---

9   The *Upanishads* are written philosophical thoughts of enlightened beings that primarily focus on spiritual enlightenment, and were written circa 700–400 BCE.
10 This classic yogic text was composed by Svatmarama in the 15th century as a compilation of the earlier *Hatha* yoga texts. Svatmarama incorporates older Sanskrit concepts into his synthesis. It runs in the line of *Hindu Yoga* (as opposed to Buddhist and Jain traditions) and is dedicated to Lord Shiva, the Hindu god of destruction and renewal.

time, those at the consciousness level above can recognize and understand people from the same level and all lower levels. However, they cannot understand people at the higher level of consciousness. Therefore, the responsibility of each yoga practitioner is to work tirelessly on expanding their level of consciousness, through developing their awakened awareness.

It is important for us, as yoga practitioners and therapists, to understand all aspects of spirituality in the context of our own growth as well as to understand where our clients are. Our own spiritual intelligence and spiritual competency grants us the ability to recognize spiritual distress, spiritual pain, and the spiritual needs of our clients. Thus, it opens the possibility of providing appropriate individual spiritual care to our clients.

The daily yogic *sadhana* invites the journey of self-discovery and allows for facing our shadow, bringing unprocessed experiences into our consciousness. It fosters self-acceptance and paves the way to profound personal transformation. This process can be very challenging and difficult at the beginning, and is not for the faint hearted. Facing our own warts and mistakes may be ego-shattering, and requires grit and a lot of courage.

The personal experience and transformation brought about by daily yogic practices develop, in turn, our own spiritual intelligence and competence. Such personal experience of a variety of yogic practices allows the yoga therapist to recommend an effective protocol for their client, resulting in their spiritual transformation and improvement of their well-being and health. Our own *sadhana* also increases our own sensitivity of our five senses and beyond, expanding our ability to assess the state of our clients. Therefore, daily *sadhana* should be understood as our core competency. Such practice enables us to strive for all the qualities, as mentioned by Joseph LePage, founder and director of Integrative Yoga Therapy (quoted with the author's permission):

QUALITIES OF A YOGA THERAPIST

An appropriate analogy for Yoga therapy is a bird whose two wings must move in synchrony in order for the Yoga healing process to unfold optimally. One wing is a thorough understanding of the tools, techniques and methodologies. The other wing is the vision of Yoga therapy as a lifelong journey of healing, both for the therapist and for the care receiver. This second wing is supported by the cultivation of essential qualities, such as careful listening. It is the integration of these qualities, along with an in-depth knowledge of the techniques that allow the Yoga therapist to practice authentically.

The following is an elaboration of these qualities:

Selfless service: *nihsvaartha seva*
The Yoga therapist receives fair compensation for professional services, but also cultivates an attitude of selfless service; a vision of healing larger than their own personal goals, wants and needs. Through this expanded vision, the therapist becomes an embodiment of healing to their clients, the community and ultimately to all humanity.

Grounding: *dṛḍhatā*
The Yoga therapist cultivates grounding and stability at all levels of being. This begins with the physical body where they develop the strength and stability to assist with poses confidently. Grounding extends to the psycho-emotional level, where our consistent practice of centering and stability allows us to meet challenges presented by care receivers safely and confidently.

Self-healing: *svacikitsā*
The Yoga therapist upholds the inherent capacity of all care receivers to awaken their own inherent potential for self-healing. Confidence in the process of self-healing begins with the therapists themselves as they transform their own health at all dimensions of being through Yoga.

Conscious presence: *cetana upasthiti*
Conscious presence is being present in each moment, experiencing each moment as the sole reality. The Yoga therapist is aware of the past in the form of the care receiver's history as well their own patterns of conditioning. The Yoga therapist also has a vision of the future in terms of the goals for healing for the client. Yoga therapy, however, only takes place in the present moment, with the therapist fully conscious of all that is happening both within themselves and within the receiver at all levels of being. This presence is characterized by an intense curiosity in regard to the receiver's process of healing along with deep compassion as well as awareness of the constant presence of their own light of healing.

Careful listening: *śravaṇam*
In effective Yoga therapy, the therapist seldom offers advice or opinions, but listens carefully and sensitively to what their care receivers are communicating in order to respond appropriately. This listening involves careful attention to what is communicated and repetition of key points for clarity and also to allow the speaker to hear what they are expressing in a way that supports Self-knowledge. There is also a deeper level of intuitive listen which develops along the therapist's own spiritual

journey, an intuitive understanding of the human being which allows us to "see" the care receiver's entire life story and the full dimension of their needs for healing both within and beyond what they are communicating.

Skillful speech: *vāca kauśalaṃ*

Even as our listening skills deepen, we also learn to respond to what we hear more sensitively and always within the framework of the care receiver's overall journey and goals for healing. Skillful speech begins with the ability to reflect communication back to the speaker in ways that are easily received and genuinely constructive. Skillful speech continues with the ability to ask questions that lead to increased awareness on the part of the receiver rather than offering advice or suggestions. Skillful speech is also present in developing plans for healing in a way that is co-creative rather than prescriptive.

Skillful means: *upakaraṇā kauśalaṃ*

The Yoga therapist has an in-depth understanding of a wide range of the tools of Yoga therapy including *asana*, *pranayama*, *mudra*, *meditation* and *yoga nidra* as well as the philosophical and historical framework in which they evolved. The therapist also has an in-depth understanding of anatomy, physiology and kinesiology in relation to the effects and benefits of these tools. Furthermore, the Yoga therapist has an understanding of disease processes both from a Western and an Ayurvedic perspective. Skillful means is the seamless integration of all of these areas of knowledge within Yoga's light of intuitive wisdom.

Patience: *dhairya*

The healing process is unique for each individual. It cannot be rushed and, like the butterfly's wings, must unfold as part of a process in which all of the stages of healing occur naturally. The therapist must be mindful of allowing this process to unfold, never rushing forward in the name of achieving short-term goals.

Enthusiasm: *utsāha*

The Yoga therapist is familiar with all aspects of Yoga as a healing modality, but also has a natural tendency to gravitate toward a specific area or areas. A Yoga therapist who cultivates their strengths and areas of interest is passionate about their particular area of concentration, whether it be the physical body, the subtle body or the psycho-emotional body. This enthusiasm supports the care receiver in their own healing process.

Committed personal practice: *sādhanā*
A practice designed for the needs of the individual generally provides optimal healing. The most effective way for the therapist to create a personal practice for others is to develop their own consistent individual practice, and to assess carefully how it meets their needs.

Study of self and scriptures: *svādhyāya*
The Yoga therapist facilitates care receivers in widening their perspectives of themselves and life as a whole, which is one of the most important dimensions of healing. This process begins when the therapist explores areas of limitation, pain and suffering in their own lives, allowing them to effectively facilitate self-study in others. This process of self-study is grounded in an in-depth understanding of the essential sacred scriptures of Yoga including Patanjali's *Yoga Sutras*, the *Bhagavad Gita*, the *Upanishads* and the texts of *Hatha Yoga*.

Simplicity: *saralatā*
When we begin to practice Yoga therapy, there may be a tendency to offer many tools and techniques in order to provide "the most healing." For effective Yoga therapy, however, less is usually more, and offering a few tools and techniques fully and authentically is generally most helpful. This simplicity is a reflection of a growing clarity within our own journey in which we start exploring many techniques and, over time, are able to simply rest in the simplicity of our own essential nature.

Generosity: *udāratā*
The Yoga therapist maintains appropriate boundaries in terms of time and energy to avoid burnout. The therapist also introduces material at a pace that is easily accessible for the care receiver. At the same time, he or she offers all of their knowledge and understanding of Yoga generously, showing that knowledge of Yoga is universal and belongs to all of humanity. Self-knowledge is the evolutionary future of humanity.

Compassion: *karuṇa*
Compassion is seeing clearly that all beings seek happiness and avoid suffering with the limits of their understanding. Most seek it only in the material world through achieving what they like and avoiding what they dislike. As Yoga therapists, we honor this starting point compassionately, recognizing that we, too, have sought happiness and through our surroundings but, over time, through the light of Yoga, have come to see that we are the very happiness we seek. By honoring both the

starting point and the process, we are able to see that everyone, including ourselves, is on a journey of healing. For some, the journey is predominantly directed toward physical healing while, for others, it is emotional, while all eventually come to see that ultimate healing in reunion with our true Being as a reflection of the Divine Intelligence at the heart of all things. Seeing all of us together on a single healing journey is the essence of compassion.

Witness consciousness: *sākṣitva*

In Yoga therapy, a wide range of feelings, emotions and sensations, both positive and negative, may arise in the care receiver. The Yoga therapist witnesses these feelings in the receiver nonjudgmentally, creating a space where they can be expressed and integrated. The Yoga therapist creates this space for the care receiver at the level of the physical body, the mind and emotions as well as spiritually, employing skill and sensitivity to support the process while allowing the receiver's process to unfold in their own time and way. Any inclination to help the poor butterfly by forcing its wings open can result in an inability to fly fully and autonomously in later stages of the process. Even as the therapist supports witness consciousness in the care receiver, they also deepen this skill in relation to their own thoughts, feelings and core beliefs that arise within the therapy process.

Equanimity: *samatva*

Equanimity is one of the most important results of our deepening ability to witness consciously and consistently. For it is this consistent witnessing that reveals the *vasanas*, the deep core beliefs that keep us from recognizing our true inner Being whose very nature is equanimity. With growing equanimity, we are able to rest in the calm depths of our inner being regardless of what is happening at the surface level of sensations, thoughts and feelings that arise in Yoga therapy and in daily living.

Integrity: *arjava*

An essential facet of integrity in Yoga therapy is standing in our authenticity as healers within the vision of Yoga where health is integration of body, mind and Spirit within a growing understanding that our true Being is inherently whole and complete. In this spirit, we offer Yoga therapy as optimal Yoga practices for individual needs as a vehicle for healing at all levels of being, rather than prescribing specific yoga techniques to cure disease. Integrity is also recognizing when we are able to work with a receiver effectively, and when it is appropriate to refer the person to another care provider or Yoga therapist with a particular specialization.

Multidimensional awareness: *pañca kośa darśana*

The Yoga therapist holds a vision of the whole person so that even if they're focusing on the physical body, they are also seeing, sensing and responding to their receiver's needs at the energetic, psycho-emotional, wisdom, and spiritual levels. This multidimensional perspective, framed within the model of the five *koshas*, naturally cultivates greater awareness within the therapist of all the dimensions involved in healing. The five *koshas* model also brings awareness to each of these dimensions within the care receiver, naturally opening them to multidimensional healing.

Intuition: *nidhyāna*

The Yoga therapist has a wide range of tools and techniques for assessing the receiver's needs, and a theoretical and technical understanding of these is essential for the practice of Yoga therapy. Beyond this technical understanding, intuition plays an important role in knowing how and when to employ these tools and techniques in the care receiver's journey. Intuition expresses itself through an inner knowing that arises spontaneously from within the therapist in silent communion with our own inner being.

Creativity: *pratibhā*

Yoga therapy is an art and a science, and with each group or individual we meet, we learn and teach something in a completely new way. This openness to Yoga therapy as a field of infinite possibilities allows for tremendous creativity, keeping our teaching fresh, alive, and relevant to each receiver's individual needs. Creativity is especially relevant in relation to those who practice and teach *Hatha Yoga* in that the spirit of creativity, alongside the maintenance of tradition, was at the heart of the *Hatha Yoga* renaissance in the 1920s. Many of the aspects of this renaissance, including Yoga instruction to householders including women and various castes, was a completely unique and creative adaptation of Yoga to the needs of modern life.

Self-nourishment: *Atma poṣaṇa*

We will be able to nourish others only to the extent that we are able to nourish ourselves. This self-nourishment is multidimensional within the model of the five *koshas*. We nourish the physical body with optimal diet, lifestyle and daily Yoga practice. We also receive body work and other healing techniques to keep the importance of the therapeutic relationship always in view. At the level of the energy body, the therapist avails themselves of subtle body healing techniques to balance the *chakras*, ensure the optimal flow of the *pranavayus*, and balance the *nadis*, so that sun and moon are harmonized appropriately, allowing us to abide in equanimity more consistently. Energetic nourishment is also supported by regular connection to nature and sources of pure energy.

At the psycho-emotional level, we nourish ourselves through rest and stress management in the form of regular *yoga nidra* and other relaxation practices. We also set time aside for play and exploring life's mysteries. At the wisdom level, we gradually reduce our identification with negative core beliefs and tendencies that cause tension and disharmony, thereby releasing us from the inner and outer conflict that keep us from nourishing ourselves with positive thoughts, feelings, beliefs and activities. At the bliss level, the release from negativity allows us to nourish ourselves with positive thoughts and energy that reflect our true Being, allowing us to align with the Divine Source Energy, the very essence of nourishment. As we nourish ourselves, we support our own process of inner healing and can model this multidimensional healing for our clients through our words and through our energetic presence.

Gratitude: *kṛtajñāta*

Gratitude is recognizing life, including its challenges, as a precious gift, a rare and unique opportunity for appreciation and learning. This recognition of life's inherent value supports us in accepting and embracing every experience as it presents itself in each moment, allowing each human being to refine and unfold their unique talents and possibilities. By modeling this quality for our care receivers, we open them to the possibility of unfolding their own unique possibilities, which is an essential facet of healing.

Inner freedom: *kaivalya*

Kaivalya literally means aloneness, but in the context of Yoga therapy, it can be translated as absolute autonomy through freedom from all the conditioned beliefs that form the limited personality. It is this autonomy that allows us to clearly recognize our absolute unity with all of creation, and from that unity, to interact ongoingly in a spirit of compassion, peace, and harmony. *Kaivalya* allows us to live and work with a sense of lightness and ease and to see and serve our care receivers with compassion, enthusiasm, and objectivity, optimally supporting their journey of healing.

Surrender: *praṇidhāna*

Surrender is the recognition that there is an all-encompassing intelligence at the heart of creation that guides our life journey. This intelligence has inspired us to embark on our own journey of Yoga healing and to share to with others through Yoga therapy. As we align with this source energy, we are naturally guided to complete our own process of healing and to support others on their journey.

Faith: *śraddha*

Faith is the absolute knowing that Yoga is a process of transformation that has healed us at all levels of being. We also have faith that Yoga has the power and potential to heal all those we receive through offering optimal techniques for healing to each care receiver we meet.

WORDS OF WISDOM

Here is what one of the yoga therapy community elders, founder of iRest, and psychotherapist Richard Miller says about the importance of *sadhana* for yoga teachers and therapists:

> I would say *sadhana* is critical, because it's driven by a deep urge that we all have within us, to what I would call enlightenment. We have the need for food, clothing, shelter, and social aspects. We also have an enlightenment urge to basically become all that we're destined or capable of being. That urge was early on in my teens. In my 20s I was fortunate to meet a mentor who met me in that drive. When I began working with clients with her, that understanding was part of the work that we were doing.
>
> One of the things I think is very important for yoga therapists in particular is the understanding that the client is none other than ourself in their own form. We're both expressions of an essential nature out of which we took birth. We're not helping the client to become whole. We're helping them recognize their existing wholeness and then grow into that. I would say we help to clear away the obstructions that are preventing them from abiding in that.
>
> Yoga therapists oftentimes come with the intention to change, to fix, or alter their students or their clients. I think they need to understand that in each of us there is the same part, which doesn't need to be fixed, altered, or changed, but awakened to. Then we can address what's in the body and the mind that may need altering.
>
> The first thing that I will do with the client or with the student, or when I'm

teaching, is to introduce them to that core, felt sense of wholeness. Recognize it and then we keep using it as a touchstone. I can help the yoga therapy student or client I am working with touch it fairly quickly. To become established in it is a whole long process, because of all the tendencies, the habits, and the psychological issues (*samskaras*) obscure it. But at least they've had a glimpse. This deep spiritual stuff is an essence of yoga.

However, many yoga therapy programs tend to objectify the person, like in medical care. The doctors are coming into room 306 and seeing the broken leg. Yoga therapists are coming into room 209, and seeing the neck that needs to be fixed, or the bad back that needs to be helped, or the depression that needs to be fixed, or anxiety that needs to be overcome.

I think it is also very important that yoga therapists recognize their limitations. Their ability to say "I would love for you to talk to such and such person about this" when they see the client may have a glimpse and describing it to them.

This is where *sadhana* and humility comes in. We need to learn to recognize and respect what we don't know and have yet to understand, and that we're growing constantly into deeper understandings. If we can admit that, then we can seek advice. We're in trouble if we don't recognize our own limitations or can't admit to them.

Stephanie Lopez talks about "sitting with the other" in these words:

We see the whole person. That's a yogic perspective. The essence of sitting with, is that I no longer see them as a separate, the other, that needs to be fixed and changed.

I use the wisdom gained through my own experience. It comes out of the deep listening and meeting someone heart to heart rather than "me to you." We move from seeing another person as the other, another body sitting across from us, into feeling the deep connection on the level of the essence we both share. That is what can be discovered or revealed through *sadhana*.

Through *sadhana* one may understand that although paradoxical, both connections are true and possible. Recognizing that there is some mystery here, that the underlying essence giving rise to the person in front of me is in myself as well. The same essence that's giving rise to the tree, to the lake, to the sky, to everything. The beauty of it is that it doesn't in any way negate the fact my eyes see the other person in front of me. This paradox seems to be natural—I see in front of me a separate person…and yet I know and feel that on the deeper level we are one and the same.

Through *sadhana* we can connect to our own essence, into our own depth.

Through firsthand experience of our own depth comes the recognition. That experience allows us to connect also to the depth of the other person. It may happen through *sadhana* or, on a rare occasion, it may come in the form of direct spontaneous recognition. *Sadhana* helps us to stabilize that recognition. It helps us with spiritual honesty and integrity. *Sadhana* helps us to integrate these experiences of recognition and accelerates the process of maturation. So that we act in service of the deepest truth, not in service of the ego.

Some yoga teachers and yoga therapists think of *sadhana* as part of their course study. When they graduate the program, they think of *sadhana* as an optional tool of self-care. Little do they realize that *sadhana* offers an opportunity for self-discovery, for uncovering and assimilating the parts of ourselves we couldn't face in the past. Such a journey grows our compassion for ourselves and for others; it expands our consciousness and miraculously grows the peace and joy within. This inner work does not end when we graduate yoga teacher training or yoga therapy training. It must continue throughout our professional life, because it becomes our core competency.

WHAT IS THE DIFFERENCE BETWEEN YOGA THERAPIST AND YOGA TEACHER?

Many yoga therapists have difficulties formulating the difference between yoga therapy and yoga teachers or practitioners of other alternative approaches to health and healing. Here are some points that can be considered when we think of the uniqueness of yoga therapy.

Direct experience of yogic tools

Yoga therapy emphasizes the importance of personal practice and the direct experience of practitioners. This approach of "living what we preach" provides several key benefits. By maintaining a consistent personal practice, yoga therapists gain firsthand experience with the tools and techniques they recommend to clients. This direct experience allows them to:

- Speak authentically about the effects and benefits of various practices
- Provide nuanced guidance based on their own challenges and insights
- Demonstrate a genuine commitment to the principles they teach
- Develop a more profound understanding of yogic concepts and practices
- Experience the subtle effects of different techniques over time

- Refine their ability to adapt practices for individual needs.

A consistent *sadhana* supports the ongoing development and well-being of the therapist by:

- Providing a foundation for self-reflection and personal transformation
- Offering tools for managing stress and maintaining balance
- Fostering a deeper connection to the spiritual aspects of yoga
- Being fully present and attuned to clients during sessions
- Accessing intuitive insights that can benefit their therapeutic approach.

This approach of "living what we preach" not only enhances the effectiveness of yoga therapy but also maintains the integrity of the tradition.

Embodied awareness

Embodied awareness is indeed a fundamental aspect of yoga therapy. This approach integrates the mind and body, fostering a deep connection with our physical sensations, emotions, and thoughts in the present moment. It goes beyond mere physical exercise, emphasizing the quality of attention brought to each practice. This mindful approach becomes a form of "moving meditation," allowing practitioners to fully tune into their bodies and gauge appropriate responses.

While embodied awareness offers numerous benefits, it's important to approach the practice with care while working with clients:

- For individuals with trauma history, intense body awareness may initially be overwhelming, so a gradual, trauma-informed approach is crucial.
- Be mindful of the difference between embodied awareness and dissociation, which can sometimes be mistaken for spiritual connection.
- Find the right balance between focused attention and relaxation, to avoid strain or tension.

Embodied awareness is a powerful tool for enhancing the yoga therapy experience. By bringing full attention to the present moment and cultivating a deep connection with the body, practitioners can unlock profound benefits for both physical and mental well-being. By teaching the client mindfulness we move the practice into a holistic approach for cultivating presence, self-awareness, and overall health.

Daily inner work through *sadhana*

Sadhana is the cornerstone of yoga therapy and personal growth. This consistent inner work forms the foundation of transformation, allowing practitioners to cultivate awareness, balance, and spiritual connection. *Sadhana* is more than just a routine; it's a sacred commitment to oneself. This daily practice serves as an anchor, grounding us in our spiritual journey amidst the chaos of everyday life. The beauty of *sadhana* lies in its flexibility and its ability to evolve with the practitioner.

The power of *sadhana* comes from its regularity. By practicing daily, preferably at the same time and place, we create a rhythm that aligns our body, mind, and spirit. This consistency helps to:

- Establish a strong mind–body connection
- Cultivate discipline and willpower
- Create a sacred space in our daily lives.

As we grow and change, so, too, does our *sadhana*. What begins as a structured set of *asanas* or meditation techniques may transform over time. This evolution is natural and should be embraced, as it reflects our personal growth and changing needs.

As we deepen our practice, a subtle shift occurs:

- Initial stage, doing: In the beginning, *sadhana* may feel like a task. We consciously set aside time to "do" our practice, often focusing on the physical aspects and tangible results.

- Intermediate stage, integrating: With time, elements of our practice begin to permeate our daily life. We might find ourselves naturally aware of our breath during a stressful meeting or silently repeating a mantra while commuting.

- Advanced stage, being: Eventually, the line between "practice" and "life" blurs. The awareness cultivated through mindfulness extends throughout our day. The compassion developed through *seva* becomes our natural response to others. We move from "doing yoga" to "living yoga" and finally to "being in the state of yoga."

One of the profound effects of consistent *sadhana* is the gradual transformation of our desires:

- Reduction of material cravings: As we connect more deeply with our inner self, the pull of external possessions and achievements often diminishes.
- Shift in priorities: What once seemed important may lose its allure. We may find greater joy in simple pleasures and spiritual pursuits.
- Cultivation of contentment: Regular practice helps us develop *santosha* (contentment), reducing the constant craving for more.

As our practice deepens, we learn the subtle art of surrendering:

- Letting go of control: We begin to trust in a higher power or the natural flow of life (*Ishvara pranidhana*).
- Acceptance: Rather than fighting against what is, we learn to accept and work with our current reality.
- Flow state: We move from rigid self-discipline to a more fluid state of being, where our practice feels effortless and joyful.

In conclusion, *sadhana* is a powerful tool for personal transformation. Through consistent practice, we cultivate awareness, reduce attachments, and move towards a state of being, where every moment becomes an opportunity for spiritual growth. As we progress on this path, we find that the peace and clarity we experience during our formal practice begin to infuse every aspect of our lives, leading to a more balanced, joyful, and purposeful existence.

Multilayered approach to the client using the *pancha koshas* framework

Yoga therapy indeed offers a uniquely comprehensive approach to healing and wellness, drawing from the ancient wisdom of Ayurveda and the holistic understanding of human existence. The *pancha koshas* framework, which forms the foundation of this approach, provides a multidimensional perspective on health and well-being that sets yoga therapy apart from many other alternative healthcare modalities.

The *pancha koshas* model describes five interconnected layers of human existence:

- *Annamaya kosha* (physical body): Yoga therapy employs specific *asanas* (postures) and movement practices to address physical imbalances and promote overall health. These practices can help increase flexibility, strengthen muscles, and improve overall physical function. When performed with mindfulness and breathing techniques, the practices impact all layers of human existence.

- *Pranamaya kosha* (energy body): Through *pranayama* (breathwork) and other energy-balancing techniques, yoga therapy works to optimize the flow of *prana* throughout the body. This can help improve respiratory health and overall vitality.

- *Manomaya kosha* (mental-emotional body): Yoga therapy incorporates meditation, mindfulness practices, and specific postures known to influence mood and mental states. These techniques can help reduce stress, anxiety, and depression while promoting emotional balance.

- *Vijnanamaya kosha* (wisdom body): By encouraging self-reflection and cultivating awareness, yoga therapy helps individuals tap into their inner wisdom and intuition. This can lead to better decision-making and a deeper understanding of oneself.

- *Anandamaya kosha* (bliss body): While not imposing any specific spiritual beliefs, yoga therapy recognizes the importance of connecting with our inner essence or higher self. Practices that foster this connection can promote a sense of purpose, meaning, and overall well-being.

The integration of yoga therapy with Ayurvedic principles further enhances its holistic nature. Ayurveda provides a framework for understanding individual constitutions (*doshas*) and how they relate to health and imbalance. This allows yoga therapists to tailor their approach to everyone's unique needs, addressing imbalances across all five *koshas* in a personalized manner that few other modalities can match.

Continuous effort on raising consciousness

The continuous effort to raise our consciousness is indeed a defining characteristic of yoga therapy that sets it apart from many other complementary practices. This commitment to personal growth and self-realization not only enhances the therapist's effectiveness but also directly impacts the therapeutic relationship and the client's healing journey.

The pursuit of higher consciousness is a core aspect of yoga therapy:

- Meditation practices: Engaging in various forms of meditation to cultivate awareness and connect with deeper levels of consciousness.
- Spiritual inquiry: Exploring existential questions and seeking to understand the nature of reality and the self.
- Energy work: Practicing techniques to refine and balance the subtle energy body, such as working with *chakras* and *nadis*.

This ongoing work on consciousness significantly influences the therapeutic relationship:

- Authenticity: Therapists can speak from direct experience, offering genuine insights and guidance.
- Empathy and compassion: Deeper self-understanding fosters greater empathy and compassion for clients.
- Energetic resonance: The therapist's elevated consciousness can create a supportive energetic field for the client's growth.

The focus on consciousness distinguishes yoga therapy by:

- Addressing root causes: Looking beyond symptoms to understand deeper patterns and imbalances.
- Promoting self-healing: Empowering clients to tap into their innate healing capacities.
- Integrating mind, body, and spirit: Offering a truly holistic approach that acknowledges the interconnectedness of all aspects of being.

In conclusion, the continuous effort to raise consciousness is a fundamental aspect of yoga therapy that profoundly influences both the therapist and the therapeutic process. This commitment to personal growth and the self-realization of the yoga therapist creates a unique healing environment that supports clients in reconnecting with their inner selves and accessing their own transformative potential. It is this dedication to consciousness that truly sets yoga therapy apart as a powerful tool for holistic healing and personal evolution.

In addition, we invite yoga therapists to review a comprehensive work by many experts published in the *International Journal of Yoga Therapy 24* (2014) titled "Yoga Therapy: The Profession," available on the IAYT's website.[11] It offers many

---

11   https://meridian.allenpress.com/ijyt/issue/24/1

perspectives on the new emerging yoga therapy profession as well as the qualities of yoga therapists.

OPPORTUNITIES FOR YOGA THERAPISTS IN HEALTHCARE

We have already mentioned that interest has grown globally in identifying factors that may contribute to healthy aging and longevity. Key aspects of the role that spirituality may play in promoting healthy aging include increased social support, associations with improved quality of life, decreased mortality and reduction of some of the chronic conditions discussed, psychological and mental health and resilience, purpose in life, improved cognitive function, and better management of end-of-life and issues around death.[12,13]

However, while there may be some correlations between spirituality and health outcomes, there is no "one-size-fits-all" approach to spirituality. It is essential to remember that there are significant differences in terms of sex, ethnicity, cultural background, education, and characteristics of family nuclei and communities regarding the interpretation of the role that spirituality can play in improving the health of the patient. This may generate profound difficulties in the application of spiritual interventions.

In previous chapters we mentioned that while medical staff recognize the importance of spiritual care, due to lack of time, they rely mostly on chaplains to deliver this care. However, as the research shows, spirituality remains an often neglected component of caregiving in serious illnesses.[14] Another international study in 2008 surveyed over 4000 nurses and found that spiritual care was very rarely provided.[15] In addition, only about 54 percent of hospitals in the USA had chaplains on their staff.[16]

---

12 Dezutter, J., Casalin, S., Wachholtz, A., Luyckx, K., Hekking, J., and Vandewiele, W. (2013) "Meaning in life: An important factor for the psychological well-being of chronically ill patients?" *Rehabilitation Psychology 58*, 4, 334–341. doi: 10.1037/a0034393.

13 Niu, Y., McSherry, W., and Partridge, M. (2020) "An understanding of spirituality and spiritual care among people from Chinese backgrounds: A grounded theory study." *Journal of Advanced Nursing 76*, 10, 2648–2659. doi: 10.1111/jan.14474.

14 Balboni, T. A. and Balboni, M. J. (2018) "The spiritual event of serious illness." *Journal of Pain and Symptom Management 56*, 5, 816–822. doi: 10.1016/j.jpainsymman.2018.05.018.

15 Taylor, E. J., Pariñas, S., Mamier, I., Atarhim, M. A., *et al.* (2023) "Frequency of nurse-provided spiritual care: An international comparison." *Journal of Clinical Nursing 32*, 3–4, 597–609. doi: 10.1111/jocn.16497.

16 Cadge, W., Freese, J., and Christakis, N. (2008) "The provision of hospital chaplaincy in the United States: A national overview." *Southern Medical Journal 101*, 6, 626–630. doi: 10.1097/SMJ.0b013e3181706856.

This may be a great opportunity for yoga therapists to fill this void. Yoga therapy may be best suited to contribute in this field since the essence of its methodology is an individual approach to each client. As yoga therapists we are required to walk our own spiritual path through daily *sadhana*. This gives us a personal experience of spiritual transformation. It also helps us to understand the importance of becoming spiritual care generalist.

Here is a list of skills we can learn to provide spiritual care and guidance to our clients.

THE SPIRITUAL CARE GENERALIST?[17]

- *Connect with your sense of spirituality, meaning, and purpose.* Through daily yoga *sadhana* and *svadyaya* we become aware and cultivate our own spirituality.

- *Acknowledge spiritual care as a core component of the yoga therapist relationship and holistic care.* Part of the clinician's responsibility is to assess a client's spiritual needs. Spiritual care can help clients cope with serious illness by finding meaning in their experience, staying connected to themselves and their community. When we acknowledge the spiritual needs of the client and family by taking the time to listen to what gives their lives meaning and what they are most afraid of, these moments can affirm our shared humanity and teach us about ourselves.

- *Cultivate intentional presence.* Noticing and practicing letting go of our judgments, as well as embracing our personal fears of illness and death, can allow us to have a more balanced perspective and be more fully available to address the needs of our client and their family. By creating time to acknowledge the importance of our own well-being, we can become more aware of how our feelings shape our care. Authentic presence also involves being open to whatever emerges, without judgment or assumptions.

- *Practice compassion.* Evidence supports the positive effects of compassion

---

17 Adopted from Miller, M., Addicott, K., and Rosa, W. E. (2023) "Spiritual care as a core component of palliative nursing." *The American Journal of Nursing 123*, 2, 54–59. doi: 10.1097/01.NAJ.0000919748.95749.e5.

on client-reported outcomes, such as an increased sense of responsibility and control over their health, increased trust in relationships with providers, and improvement in symptoms. Compassion is not a weak or soft emotion but rather a strength.

- *Assess spirituality and spiritual care needs regularly.* While many structured tools exist for this purpose, screening can include broad questions like, "What are your sources of spiritual strength and support?" and "How would you describe your belief system and/or spiritual practices?" This regular spiritual assessment is part of an ongoing process of building trust and communication, and it can normalize exploring various spiritual concerns.

    Nearly one-fifth of the population in the USA in 2008 reported not being religious at all. The reality is that many clients may have unique spiritual beliefs and needs, yet some will not use the word "spirituality." Phrases such as "whatever gives you strength," "what grounds you," "what helps you go through," and "what gives your life meaning" may be useful.[18] For these clients we can bring a sense of curiosity to their broader existential beliefs, their lived experiences of meaning and purpose, and the role of connection in their lives, such as with nature, important relationships, and the broader community.

- *Learn how to assess for and recognize a spiritual crisis, in the client and in yourself.* Hearing a client say, "I feel like all hope is gone," "What is there to care about?" or "What have I done to deserve this?" may mean that the client requires referral to someone who has specialist skills in spiritual care. It is also important to recognize when we are at our limits and need support. For the yoga therapist it can be hard to recognize our own transient feelings of burnout, yet these feelings may also signal a deeper level of depletion or compassion fatigue. It can be helpful to understand these signs and to know how and where to ask for help, as hard as the yoga therapist may find it.

- *Identify spiritual care resources and foster partnership with a spiritual care specialist.* It is a good idea to identify the tools and supports that are available to clients and to ourselves. This could include knowing what spiritual

---

18 Adopted from Maiko, S., Johns, S. A., Helft, P. R., Slaven, J. E., Cottingham, A. H., and Torke, A. M. (2019) "Spiritual experiences of adults with advanced cancer in outpatient clinical settings." *Journal of Pain and Symptom Management* 57, 3, 576–586.e1. doi: 10.1016/j.jpainsymman.2018.11.026.

- *Continue to update your skills of spiritual care.* Providing spiritual care to the client is a skill, just like assessing the client before suggesting a yoga protocol, and it requires practice and training. It also includes tailoring spiritual assessment to the unique client's needs and priorities, and recognizing the need for spiritual care to evolve based on changing needs. Continuing education opportunities, such as the Interprofessional Spiritual Care Education Curriculum (ISPEC©), focus on understanding spirituality.[19]

    Perhaps more important is the experiential part of the study. Having a strong daily yoga *sadhana*, which includes *svadyaya* (self-study, self-observation), is the best way of experiential learning and a self-development tool. We can only help our client to go as far as we have been ourselves on our developmental healing journey. Our own experiences inform our wisdom and sensitivity to guide our clients in their developmental healing journey.

- *Incorporate evidence-informed interventions to support spiritual well-being.* Classical yoga, as described in classical texts (such as Patanjali's *Yoga Sutras*, *Hathapradipika*, and *Yoga Vashista*), is an experiential spiritual discipline. It provides a goal as a path of self-development (enlightenment) and the means to reach this goal (*yoga sadhana*). Although yoga was never intended as a therapeutic practice, the explosion of research since the late 20th century to this day provides evidence that yogic practices have strong healing properties at all levels of human beings, including the spiritual.

- *Have a basic understanding of the spiritual beliefs/values of major faith traditions.* Due to globalization and virtual technology, we live and work in multicultural communities. It is important to study and know major faith traditions. On the other hand, the deeper one goes in yoga, the easier it gets to see the genuinely spiritual parts of any religious tradition. This gives the generalist a way to provide yoga therapy in a way that clients from specific cultures can hear.

---

19 GWish (GW Institute for Spirituality & Health) (2021) Interprofessional Spiritual Care Education Curriculum (ISPEC©). https://smhs.gwu.edu/spirituality-health/program/transforming-practice-health-settings/interprofessional-spiritual-care-education-curriculum

Remember, we're not just teaching yoga—we're guiding people on their spiritual journey while honoring their unique paths. This work requires both heart and wisdom, constantly refined through practice and experience. Through my decades of experience, I've found that these guidelines aren't just professional requirements—they're the substance of transformative healing work that honors both ancient wisdom and modern understanding.

These competencies aren't just strategies; they're the very foundation of transformative yoga therapy. They enable us to serve our clients with both professional excellence and spiritual wisdom.

SPIRITUAL ASSESSMENTS

We will now consider the issue of spiritual assessment from two different points of view, self-assessment and client assessment in healthcare.

1. Self-assessment

First, we will reflect on available self-assessments. As yoga therapists we want to understand at what level our own spiritual competency is:

- How aware of ourselves are we?
- Are we aware of our own unresolved issues that can be unconsciously brought to the table during the session with the client?
- Can we hold our own triggers in check?
- What is our own belief system, and how much does it influence our approach to our client?
- Are we able to be truly present in difficult situations?
- Are we able to hold the space for a challenging client?
- Can we see where our client is ready to move?

The ability of self-awareness is crucial in any caring profession. Understanding of what we bring into a relationship allows for proper facilitating of such relationships. Our awareness of our own spiritual and existential views on life and death allows for full support of the client's spiritual views and assisting in their spiritual distress.

But perhaps, most importantly, we should understand the art of yoga therapy, which is:

- Forgetting our own tendency to "fix" anything: We are not the healers—we are only facilitating our client's self-healing.

- Listening for the meaning of the moment—what are our client's hopes?
- Meeting the client where they are, walking always half a step behind them, watching which direction they want to go in and when they are ready to move forward.
- Understanding that the personal spirituality of the caregiver affects the quality of care provided.[20]

The beauty of yoga therapy lies in its unique paradox: while its foundational wisdom and philosophical principles remain constant, the application must be highly personalized. This is similar to how a master chef uses the same basic ingredients but creates different dishes based on specific needs and circumstances.

These specific needs may vary from session to session. Personal limitations and circumstances may change. The current physical and mental state might be different. Individual goals and aspirations may shift. Daily life demands and constraints may alter, as well as readiness for specific practices differing, and this all needs constant consideration. This dynamic approach ensures that yoga therapy remains both authentic to its roots and relevant to each individual's unique journey of healing and transformation.

Here is a standardized Spiritual Supporter Scale[21] that was designed to assess the competency of the provision of spiritual care including knowledge, sensitivity to spiritual needs, and spiritual support skills. This can be used by all those engaged in a caregiving role. The scale runs from 1 = do not agree to 4 = strongly agree. The higher the number the higher the competency in provision of spiritual care, including knowledge, sensitivity to spiritual needs, and spiritual support skills.

1. Forgiveness is one of the dimensions of spirituality	1	2	3	4
2. Spirituality is related to the sphere of inner human life	1	2	3	4
3. When someone is suffering, I find it difficult to show compassion	1	2	3	4
4. The presence of loved one gives my life meaning	1	2	3	4
5. When working with another person I should consider the spiritual issues experienced by that person	1	2	3	4

---

20 Deluga, A., Dobrowolska, B., Jurek, K., Ślusarska, B., Nowicki, G., and Palese, A. (2020) "Nurses' spiritual attitudes and involvement—Validation of the Polish version of the Spiritual Attitude and Involvement List." *PLoS One* 15, 9, e0239068. doi: 10.1371/journal.pone.0239068.

21 Adopted from Fopka-Kowalczyk, M., Best, M., and Krajnik, M. (2023) "The Spiritual Supporter Scale as a new tool for assessing spiritual care competencies in professionals: Design, validation, and psychometric evaluation." *Journal of Religion and Health* 62, 2081–2111. https://doi.org/10.1007/s10943-022-01608-3

6. My relationship with God is the essence of my spiritual life	1	2	3	4
7. I believe prayer helps me in life	1	2	3	4
8. I know how to be truly present with the suffering person	1	2	3	4
9. I know that my life experiences make it difficult for me to maintain balance and spiritual peace	1	2	3	4
10. I try to be present with a person who is experiencing the feeling of hopelessness	1	2	3	4
11. Each helper should be able to provide holistic care to the client in need of support rather than only care for the physical aspects	1	2	3	4
12. I need other people to be present in the situation when I see no meaning in my life	1	2	3	4
13. I think that talking about spiritual problems makes people stronger and gives them power to cope with adversities such as illness or crisis	1	2	3	4
14. When I lose hope that presence of another person helps me get through this and find hope again	1	2	3	4
15. When someone wants to talk about things important to them in life, I am eager to listen	1	2	3	4
16. I think that focusing on spiritual problems takes hope away	1	2	3	4
17. Being a member of a group or community gives me strength in my life	1	2	3	4
18. I can talk to another person about their spiritual difficulties	1	2	3	4
19. In a relationship with a client in need of support, not only the body and physical symptoms but also the actual spiritual suffering and dilemmas are important	1	2	3	4
20. I can nurture my own spirituality	1	2	3	4
21. I can tell when someone is suffering on the spiritual level, for example, because they find it hard to forgive	1	2	3	4
22. When a person asks me to pray with them, I do it	1	2	3	4
23. I think it is important to give meaning to what you do in life	1	2	3	4
24. Sometimes I suggest to a client that we pray together	1	2	3	4
25. I don't know what to do when someone expects me to pray with them	1	2	3	4
26. I avoid confiding in other people	1	2	3	4
27. I have enough of my own problems to deal with other people's spiritual pain	1	2	3	4
28. I can feel when someone is suffering and going through difficult moments	1	2	3	4
29. I can see the suffering of another person in their body language	1	2	3	4

Another excellent tool for spiritual self-assessment is offered by the European Union's Erasmus program, the Spiritual Care Competency Self-Assessment Tool©.[22] This tool was developed from the Spiritual Care Education Standard, which can be found on the EPICC (Enhancing Nurses' and Midwives' Competence in Providing Spiritual Care through Innovative Education and Compassionate Care) Network's website.[23] It allows for evaluation of the level of knowledge, skills, and attitudes in four key areas of competencies for spiritual care:

- Intrapersonal spirituality
- Interpersonal spirituality
- Spiritual care assessment and planning
- Spiritual care intervention and evaluation.

2. Client assessment in healthcare

If we are to help our clients with spiritual issues, we need to understand and assess their spiritual state. This may be challenging for several reasons. First, we should be aware of our client's cultural context or religious tradition. Some cultures do not welcome discussions on spirituality. For some clients, "spirituality" may be an "uncomfortable" word. Yet these conversations may play an important role in our client's health and they need to happen. We, as yoga therapists, need to be able to facilitate such conversations if we are to be effective in helping our clients.

Being aware of spiritual experience doesn't mean ability to define it. Often spirituality means experiencing ambiguity and struggle. Each person is the expert of their life's journey. We can help them recognize and explore and sometimes help them reframe their uniqueness through listening. We can hold space for them and offer silence as presence, not an emptiness to be filled. We can also be aware of the need to *be with* and to *bear painful feelings* as we grow in our ability to *be present* with another.

In research we notice two broad approaches to spiritual assessment. In religious studies the approach has been somewhat limited to a specific religion (mostly Christian in North America). In healthcare the assessment has a "one-size-fits-all" approach. Even so, many new assessment tools were proposed

---

22 https://research.tilburguniversity.edu/en/publications/spiritual-care-in-palliative-care-working-towards-an-eapc-task-fo

23 www.epicc-network.org

in healthcare after 2000. In 2007, Katerndahl and Oyiriaru proposed the Biopsychosocialspiritual Model,[24] which had the following items on the Spiritual Symptom Scale:

- Peacefulness
- A reason for living
- Your life has been productive
- Peace of mind
- Sense of purpose
- Able to reach down deep into yourself for comfort
- Sense of harmony within yourself.

Soon after this, new tools were created, such as the Hospice Outcomes and Patient Evaluation (HOPE)[25] and FICA,[26] a spiritual history tool. The acronym FICA comes from:

- *Faith*, belief, meaning:
    - Do you consider yourself to be spiritual?
    - What gives your life meaning?

- *Importance* and influence:
    - What importance does spirituality has in your life?

- *Community:*
    - Is your community of support to you? How?

- *Action* in care:
    - How would you like me, as your healthcare provider, to address spiritual issues in your healthcare?

All these can be used to elicit a meaningful discussion with your client. However,

---

24 Katerndahl, D. and Oyiriaru, D. (2007) "Assessing the Biopsychosociospiritual Model in primary care: Development of the Biopsychosociospiritual Inventory (BioPSSI)." *The International Journal of Psychiatry in Medicine 37*, 4. doi: 10.2190/PM.37.4.d.
25 Centers for Medicare & Medicaid Services (no date) "HOPE." www.cms.gov/medicare/quality/hospice/hope
26 Puchalski, C. M. (2013) "The FICA Spiritual History Tool #274." *Journal of Palliative Medicine 17*, 1, 105–106. doi: 10.1089/jpm.2013.9458.

as mentioned, these tools have a "one-size-fits-all" approach and do not take into account individual cases with their cultural, educational, and beliefs system aspects. In "The relationship between spirituality and health outcomes,"[27] Aligh, Daniel, and Halina note some challenges in measuring the influence of spirituality on health outcomes.

Spirituality is a complex and multifaceted construct, making its measurement challenging. There is no universally agreed-upon definition or measurement tool for spirituality, leading to variations in how it is assessed across studies. Different measures may capture different aspects of spirituality, making comparisons and generalizations difficult. Studies examining spirituality often rely on self-report measures, which are subject to biases. Participants may provide socially desirable responses or have difficulty accurately reporting their spiritual beliefs, experiences, or practices.

While there is evidence for a positive relationship between spirituality and health, the science has yet to determine whether spirituality directly influences health outcomes, or if other factors contribute to the observed associations. The relationship between spirituality and health outcomes may vary across different cultural, religious, and spiritual contexts. Findings from studies conducted in one population or religious group may not necessarily apply to others; it is crucial to consider the cultural and contextual factors that influence the relationship between spirituality and health.

In *Yoga Therapy as a Whole-Person Approach to Health* we dealt extensively with yogic assessment, through five *koshas*, to evaluate the client's general state of health. In what follows, we will focus on more specific ways to assess the spiritual state of the client, as per yogic philosophy. However, we need to remember that the client is One Whole and not the sum of parts, as the healthcare system stipulates.

YOGIC TOOLS FOR ASSESSMENT AND HEALTH EVALUATION[28]

Yoga has its own traditional and cultural system of assessment, diagnosis, and health evaluation. However, as it does not seem to have a "standardized tool," many in yoga therapy practice claim (mistakenly, I believe) that it doesn't have its

---

27 Alih, F., Daniel, S., and Halina, A. (2024) "The relationship between spirituality and health outcomes." www.researchgate.net/publication/378942071
28 Based on Dr. Bhavanani's contribution to our book: Majewski, L. and Bhavanani, A. (2020) *Yoga Therapy as a Whole-Person Approach to Health*. London and Philadelphia, PA: Singing Dragon.

own system. This misconception often fosters an unhealthy dependency on the modern medical diagnosis alone. We need to be clear that we cannot move out of our Scope of Practice and "borrow" assessment tools from other professions, and furthermore, it is not correct to create therapeutic yogic plans based on the results of such borrowed assessment tools. It follows that both the assessment and the therapeutic plan should be based on knowledge from the ancient texts, and should, as far as possible, merge together seamlessly.

The development of these yoga therapy tools for clinical assessment is a work in process worldwide. What we can do today is set the standards for assessment tools in the field of yoga therapy. We can show examples of this work in progress. We can encourage others to read the ancient texts and then find ways to bring this knowledge into the modern-day clinical setting. Perhaps at the end we will not be limited to one standard assessment tool. Perhaps there will be as many tools developed as the situations and environments in which the assessments take place. Nevertheless, we need to be aware of the standards and frameworks of yoga therapy in order to create adequate tools.

NEED FOR YOGIC ASSESSMENT TOOLS

Yoga therapy must never be limited to a mere treatment of an externalized diagnosis or to symptoms. Hence, it is imperative we have tools to "tailor-make" individualized protocols or modules that take into account a thorough search for the "root cause" of the disease, and then find a way out of it with awareness.

It is also important that an attempt be made to help the client understand and accept the root cause of their problem and further familiarize themselves with factors causing, aggravating, or mitigating it. The client's self-awareness is often the only way to prevent worsening of the condition and its relapse, and to facilitate self-reliant conscious measures towards healing by the client.

Of course, the inference drawn from such a detailed yogic analysis can assist us in forming a baseline for pre-treatment and post-treatment comparisons. This also acts as a reference to assess progress in therapy at various points of time in order to make modifications or advancements accordingly.

FRAMEWORK OF YOGA THERAPY

The often-quoted traditional basic framework for the application of yoga as therapy is usually based on a derivative of the teachings of Maharishi Patanjali, as codified through his *Yoga Sutras*.[29] Verses 16–26 of the second chapter (*Sadhana pada*) elaborate the concept of addressing the problem, finding its cause, and then applying the therapeutic remedy (the goal of therapy) through use of appropriate tools (*heya-hetu*; *hana-upaya*).

1. The first and foremost step in this comprehensive template of yoga therapy is to try and understand as completely as possible the nature of the problem/issue/challenge/manifest suffering (*heya*). It is important to focus on how long the problem has been in existence, how severe it is, and how it impacts the client's daily life. We need to assess together with the client the physical, emotional, mental, social, financial, and spiritual aspects, to have a holistic picture of the current "state" of the individual who is seeking our help.

2. The second step attempts to find the possible causes of the problem (*hetu*). This must not stop at a superficial level of symptoms, but try and unravel the potential root causes that are casing the manifest signs and symptoms of disease. It is important to make a complete search for internal causes, which could include genetic predisposition, maladapted stress responses, energy imbalances, distorted perceptions, as well as negative emotions and self-image. On the other hand, external causes could be infective, accidental, environmental, or traumatic in nature. Finally, we need to address in detail the role of an unhealthy lifestyle, as this is often the main cause of the whole problem. An example would be two clients with the same symptoms—both obese and both depressed. One may be depressed because they are obese, and the other may be obese because they are depressed.

3. In the third step, a joint understanding is developed between the client and

---

29 *Yoga Darshan* of Maharishi Patanjali's *Yoga Sutras* in *Sadhana pada* gives us the philosophical basis of the yoga therapy template through the concepts of *heya-hetu*; *hana-upaya*. These are derived from the following verses:
   2:16, Prevent those miseries that are yet to occur (*heyam duhkham anagatam*).
   2:17, Suffering is caused by a misunion between the observer and the observed (*drashtri drishyayoh samyogah heya hetuh*).
   2:23, This union enables us to experience and attain mastery of our true Self (*sva svami saktyoh svarupa upalabdhi hetuh samyogah*).
   2:24, This union is caused by ignorance (*tasya hetuh avidya*).
   2:25, Dissolution of ignorance breaks this union and enables emancipation (*tat abhavat samyogah abhavah hanam tat drishi kaivalyam*).
   2:26, Constant and conscious discerning intellect dissolves ignorance (*viveka khyatih aviplava hana upayah*).

the therapist towards setting the target goals for the therapeutic process (*hana*). The client may have a certain goal in mind while the therapist has another. These goals may be different, and hence a joint discussion and collaborative and realistic plan needs to be made to avoid disappointments later. An example would be a cancer patient seeking yoga therapy to enhance their energy, improve sleep, reduce fatigue, and deal with pain, while the therapist may be more focused on "preventing an occurrence of" the cancer.

4. The final step in this process is the adoption of concrete concepts and practices that then contribute to the development of a comprehensive individualized protocol (*upaya*). This is the stage where the actual tools are determined to achieve the goal set in the third stage. This may include a combination of any or all the techniques in our therapeutic toolkit, including counseling, shifts in attitude (*bhavana*), lifestyle modifications, and practices of *Ashtanga Yoga*, *Kriya Yoga*, *Hatha Yoga*, *mantras*, *yoga nidra* meditation, *pranayama*, and, most importantly, relaxation. It is only during the relaxation phase that healing truly manifests, and hence we should never forget the importance of this often-neglected aspect of yoga therapy.

UNDERSTANDING ISSUES THAT BROUGHT THE CLIENT TO YOGA THERAPY

To properly understand the client and their problem, we need to make sure that we keep our ego in check, and that we are conscious of any projections or transference that may occur as the result of our own experiences. Our own history affects our judgment, and we need to be *very* aware of this fact in order to prevent mis-assessment. Very often we have "blind spots" around our own issues, and it is always good to have some kind of mentorship set up to be able to stop our own projections getting in the way of client assessment.

In my case it manifested in a peculiar way. I noticed that after finishing the three-week intensive Beyond Cancer retreats, I would be completely depleted of energy and had to spend two to three days resting in bed, to slowly regain vitality. One day I was discussing the retreat with a friend—a yogi scholar and psychotherapist—and I mentioned this affliction. He listened carefully and then said, "Most likely you have unresolved issues around the work you are doing with cancer patients." It took only a second to realize that I have never grieved my father's death of lung cancer when I was 15. This event had happened suddenly and left me an orphan, with no support and trying to cope with PTSD. That night I let it all surface, faced it, and had a deep release. Since then I tend to be tired, which is rather to be expected after leading three weeks of intensive retreat, but never so depleted as before.

For the purpose of assessment, the five-layered existential model (*pancha koshas*) is useful as it enables us to develop a thorough understanding—through a process of observation (*darshanam*), touch (*sparshanam*), detailed interview (*prasnam*), and assessment of energy flows (*nadi pariksha*)—the issues that may be of a physical, functional, psychological, intellectual (frustrations and conflicts), or spiritual nature. In *Yoga Therapy as a Whole-Person Approach to Health* we provided a detailed assessment of *annamaya*, *pranamaya*, *manomaya*, and *vijnamaya koshas*. Here we will focus on the way to assess *anandamaya kosha*.

Many a time a client comes to us with issues that don't really seem to be discernable at the gross, physical levels. However, when we investigate deeper, we realize that something is just "not right" at a deeper level of the mind. This may be understood as the subtle root cause (*adhi*) often mentioned in yogic patho-physiology. If we set out to evaluate this "higher mind" or intellect (*buddhi*) level, we often come upon a sense of disassociation, a sense of being "out of sync" or a sense of "not being in the right place at the right time." It is as if all the different layers (*koshas*) have gone out of alignment.

The client may say that they are always late to places or events; hence they miss buses, trains, and even important appointments for job interviews. They may state that while walking down a doorway, instead of walking through the door, they end up bumping into its side frame. Many accidents are narrated where they "knew" it was "going to happen" and yet "couldn't stop it." In modern terms this may be understood as stress. Virtually every disease or disorder is caused, precipitated, or aggravated by stress.

THINGS TO LOOK FOR

After we manage to build a close and trusting relationship with our client, we need to inquire into the deeper conflicts and frustrations that are part of their life. They may not be forthcoming initially, as these are often very personal. Usually, such deeper issues start to surface only after we build a relationship of trust and gain the client's confidence. Are they at ease with themselves or not? Do they often find themselves caught in the midst of a dilemma and between a "hammer and a hard rock?" Does their conscience seem to prick a lot, and does this lead them to ruin many aspects of their life? All these are vital if we are to find the root cause of the sense of uneasiness (*dwaitham*) that is preventing our client "feeling themselves."

We need to determine if they are aware of and how well they understand their own problem and how they choose to communicate it (*vacha*). Is it more of verbal or nonverbal communication? And when we give them any suggestions, do they hear or merely listen, without hearing? How well they adapt to the stressors in their life and the choices they make are very much part of this level of existence. Are they in a reactive mode for the most part of the day, or are they responsive? Do they realize when they are reactionary and reflexive rather than responsive and reflective? All these questions enable us to understand the *vigjnanamaya kosha* aspect of our client. Unless we help them overcome and rectify any subtle imbalances at this level, with proper protocol, our mutual efforts towards healing may not be very effective.

The principles of yoga therapy involved in this part of the process are the awareness of emotions, thoughts, and choices; the calming down of the mind, focusing it inward; and the ability to fortify oneself against the omnipresent stressors. Assessment of these and of the spiritual level of existence will be possible only with time, when the relationship between the yoga professional and client grows into deep trust and mutual respect.

Each and every living being is endowed with amazing self-healing potential but are often ignorant of it. As a yoga professional, it is important that we address this and try to understand how well the client is connected to their "own Self." Are they "at ease" with themselves, or is there a sense of duality or separation between their own mind and body? Often people identify themselves with their mind—we often hear "I am my thoughts."

We need to search out the cause of their problems by addressing the core of their afflictions (the root *klesha*, *avidya*). The hold of this primary distorter of our perspective is often very tight and influences everything through ignorance. This is then compounded by the false sense of ego (*asmita*). What are the client's sources of hope, strength, and comfort? What does the client hold on to during difficult times? Do they belong to a supportive community? What things do they believe give meaning to their life? Do they believe in a greater power/god? Are they religious? Are they spiritual? What does spirituality (or religion) mean to the client? What role do their beliefs play in regaining their health? As we develop our relationship with the client, we can start such conversations. This will help us to assess this layer of existence.

The need to survive at any cost (*abhinivesha*) induces the exaggerated stress response. The diametrically opposite pulls—the attraction (*raaga*) to some things and the aversion (*dwesha*) to other things—may create deep inner conflicts. How attached are they to their likes and dislikes? Are they able to balance them or not?

Without the client's awareness and understanding of the necessity of detachment, the tranquility and equanimity of mind will remain unattainable. Only when the client realizes this can we introduce Maharishi Patanjali's concepts through the practice of self-purification (*Kriya Yoga*). The importance of discipline, self-analysis, and acceptance (*tapas, swadhyaya and Ishwar pranidhana*) as the means to overcome these afflictions may never be realized otherwise.

CONVERSATION STARTERS

As yoga professionals we must meet the client where they are, taking into account their cultural and religious background as well as their values, education, and belief system. Such a methodology can be much better tailored through conversational flow instead of a questionnaire.

The following list of questions can be great conversation starters in more conversational exploration of a client's spiritual needs.[30] You may also find it more suited to an individual approach to the client:

- Please describe the major events in last 10 years that you think might have contributed to your health challenge.
- Please describe your typical day routine (including meal times). How regular is it?
- If you were asked what belief about yourself or emotion contributed to your health challenge, what would your answer be?
- What resources have been most useful throughout your care/treatment/recovery (social, physical, mental/emotional, and spiritual)?
- What attitude would you say was most useful for you to have throughout your treatment and recovery?
- Do you struggle with any emotional issues? If so, please describe.
- What brings meaning, value, and purpose to your life?
- What lights your fire?
- Where were you before you were born? Where will you go after death?
- Have you found new meanings and values in the losses you have lived through?
- What can you create? What can you let go of?
- What is on your "bucket list" of things to do before you die?

---

30 Burhardt, M. and Nagai-Jacobson, M. G. (1985) "Dealing with spiritual concerns in the community." *Journal of Community Healing Nursing 2*, 4, 191–198.

- If you believe in the Divine, how do you name and relate to your God?

IN CONCLUSION

We, as yoga therapists, must never forget to look at the bigger picture. This can only be only with time and the trust we build with the client. If this is done efficiently and with competence, then we and the client will be able to understand the problem and its cause, and then find the remedy that needs to be applied.

To keep it short:

- Treat the client with respect, and always obtain explicit consent, especially before any hands-on examination or corrections.

- Observe the client's body, its proportions, unconscious and conscious movements, function, and their level of body awareness.

- Observe the client's breath, how slow/quick it is, and how it changes when consciousness is brought into play, such as when you ask them to breathe as opposed to when they are passively breathing.

- Listen to the client and try to understand their thoughts and expressions. Look out for the hidden aspects that may have been left unsaid.

- Gain the client's confidence and you will then find the whole "box" opens up and you get to see the real cause of the problem.

- Witness how the client relates to themself and others, and be aware of how they distort the perspective (*kleshas*). Slowly help them to also "see" this and then witness if changes occur or whether they just go into denial. If so, many more sessions may be needed.

- Put all the pieces of habitual patterns, conditioning, inherent tendencies, and latent desires together to understand where the source of the problem is. As you get to know the client better, the assessment will be shifting.

- Keep working from the gross to the subtle and to the casual, and then evaluate the changes as they manifest from the causal, through the subtle, and finally the gross levels of existence.

- Do not give up, even if it seems tough—this is the golden opportunity we have to truly help another human being out of suffering and into ease. However, always walk "half-a-step behind" the client, watching for opening to the next step.

- Be prepared that some clients may come to you to hear what they want to hear. They may not be open to any suggestions that may not be in line with their preset ideas. You may find that they have already visited a few care workers and "didn't receive any help." Very likely a solution was suggested, but they were not ready to accept it. It is up to you to evaluate how set the person is in their expectations of what they want to hear, and decide whether to continue with the sessions.

In this chapter we explored some issues connected to spirituality, which are important to yoga professionals. We stressed the significance of daily *sadhana* as a core competency for every yoga professional. We outlined the main difference between yoga therapy and other complementary disciplines. We pointed to existing opportunities for yoga professionals to provide spiritually informed yoga therapy in the healthcare system. To do this, we listed the critical competencies for yoga therapists as spiritual care generalists. And finally, we considered ways for spiritual self-assessment and how to assess the spiritual state of our clients.

In Part 2 we uncover many unusual stories from expert yoga professionals, who share their innermost experiences in their spiritual journeys. You will find that these stories reflect the importance of the points mentioned in this chapter and others in Part 1.

PART 2

FROM DARKNESS TO LIGHT

Journey of Spiritual Awakening

Introduction

If we can trust and listen to our inner divine image, or our True Self, we will act from our best, largest, kindest, most inclusive self.

RICHARD ROHR[1]

When I began exploring the profound interconnectedness of spirituality and yoga, I realized that words alone could only go so far in encapsulating the transformation such practices offer. The abstract concepts of spiritual awakening often feel intangible until they are embodied, lived, and shared through real human stories. Inspired by Paul Mills' deeply personal and impactful work, *Science, Being, & Becoming: The Spiritual Lives of Scientists*,[2] I decided to anchor this segment of the book in the lived realities of yoga practitioners and therapists whose spiritual transformations have defined their paths.

The first part of this book laid the foundations, exploring spirituality as a universal thread that transcends religion and permeates our everyday lives. Here, in this second part, I aim to give life to those principles by sharing personal stories—testimonies of courage, growth, and self-discovery. These stories illustrate how spiritual evolution, although inherent and often inevitable, is uniquely shaped by the choices we make, the challenges we endure, and the connections we foster. While spirituality may seem elusive or abstract, it becomes profoundly relatable when we hear it through the voices of those who have lived it.

A curious thing happens as we grow older. Looking back at the patterns of our lives, we begin to see an order where once we saw chaos. Random events take on meaning, spontaneous choices seem guided by some unseen hand, and the intricate weaving of life's threads reveals a purposeful design. When I reflect upon my

---

1   Rohr, R. (2019) *The Universal Christ: How a Forgotten Reality Can Change Everything We See, Hope for and Believe*. London: SPCK Publishing.
2   Mills, P. J. (2023) *Science, Being, & Becoming: The Spiritual Lives of Scientists*. Sacred Stories Publishing, LLC. Kindle Edition, p.2.

path, I often wonder: Who composed this symphony? Was it fate? My own will? The interactions with others who became unwitting co-creators of my story? Or perhaps some greater force beyond my understanding? Our lives unfold much like characters in an epic dream—whose dream we may never fully know. This mystery is a central theme in the stories I share here.

The narratives are not just about individuals but about the universal longing for transcendence, connection, and peace. They remind us that through yoga and spirituality, we can reconnect with our deepest selves, break the shackles of rigid societal expectations, and discover a vast reservoir of kindness, compassion, and wisdom within.

The stories we tell are a testament to transformation. Over the course of this project I had the privilege of interviewing over 50 long-term yoga practitioners and therapists from around the globe. Their openness and generosity in sharing their journeys left me deeply grateful and inspired. While no two paths are identical, each one bore an undeniable thread of profound inner transformation. Whether through mystical guidance, inner peace, or spirituality in action, these experiences offer vivid insights into what it means to embark on a spiritual path. All the interviewees are seasoned yoga practitioners of many years. Most of them studied and trained with teachers and gurus in India, and spent a lot of time in ashrams.

STRUCTURE AND PURPOSE: FROM INSPIRATION TO REALIZATION

Yoga, as a practice, often begins as a way to improve physical health or alleviate stress. Yet, time and again, my conversations revealed how it unfailingly evolves into something much deeper—a tool for spiritual growth, a bridge to higher consciousness, a guide toward a more compassionate existence. The practitioners and therapists I spoke with confirmed what I have long believed: spiritual development is not an optional pursuit but an innate human need. It is woven into the very fabric of our being and, when nurtured, opens us to a life of greater clarity, fulfillment, and meaning.

Through their stories, we can witness how yoga sharpens our perception, helping us see life with renewed clarity. It enables us to understand the inner self—our True Self—and transforms how we perceive the outer world. This transformation not only enhances our personal happiness but also deepens our empathy, strengthens our relationships, and enriches our professional practice as yoga therapists.

The real challenge in compiling this book was selecting which stories to include. Each narrative held a unique resonance, but to keep this volume cohesive and engaging, we chose accounts that best illustrated the rich tapestry of spiritual transformation. These stories are divided into five key chapters based on recurring themes:

- *Breaking free:* Stories of individuals liberating themselves from societal expectations, personal limitations, and internal constraints through yoga and spirituality (Chapter 7).
- *The gift of yoga:* Narratives that delve into the ways yoga became the catalyst for profound personal change (Chapter 8).
- *Inner guidance:* Accounts of mystical experiences and transformative inner dialogues that redirected lives toward purpose and meaning (Chapter 9).
- *Seeking out:* Journeys of individuals actively searching for deeper understanding and connection (Chapter 10).
- *Spirituality in action:* Stories that show spirituality as a living, breathing force embodied in acts of kindness, service, and community (Chapter 11).

Each chapter features five to seven stories, carefully condensed to preserve their essence without losing the depth of emotion and insight they carry. These accounts, although diverse in detail, resonate with universal truths—truths that may validate your own experiences or guide you on your path forward.

METHODOLOGY: A COLLABORATIVE JOURNEY

Conducting these interviews was itself a deeply rewarding process. Thanks to modern technology, geographical and time zone barriers became irrelevant as conversations unfolded over Zoom. The platform's transcript feature proved invaluable, capturing the raw authenticity of each dialogue, which was then shaped into a cohesive narrative.

In developing my interview questions, I adapted Paul Mills' original framework[3] to fit the context of yoga therapy, ensuring the conversation was both relevant and expansive. These are the questions I posed as the starters of conversation:

- Please describe any specific transpersonal, metaphysical, or mystical experiences that changed your perception of the world.

---

3 Mills, P. J. (2023) *Science, Being, & Becoming: The Spiritual Lives of Scientists*. Sacred Stories Publishing, LLC. Kindle Edition, p.2.

- How did these experiences influence your decision to become a yoga professional (or your existing practice)?
- Who were the mentors or spiritual teachers who shaped your journey?
- What challenges—personal or professional—have you faced along the way?
- How are you now sharing your insights and giving back?

The resulting stories are more than anecdotes; they are powerful testimonies of personal evolution. While not every account could be included in this volume, the ones that remain are a vibrant mosaic of the limitless possibilities that await those who embark on the spiritual path. These transformative possibilities make us better human beings.

As you read these stories, I hope you find them not only fascinating but also affirming. Perhaps they will mirror aspects of your own journey, or perhaps they will beckon you to explore new realms of understanding. At their core, these narratives aim to spark conversation and connection—encouraging us to bring spirituality into awareness in our daily lives.

The journey from darkness to light is one we all share. My hope is that this book will serve as both a guide and a companion along the way. My hope also is that the book will encourage the conversations about spirituality we tend to have avoided thus far.

CHAPTER 7

Breaking Free

Transformative journeys are described in these six personal accounts. Each weaves a compelling narrative of spiritual awakening and self-discovery through the practice of yoga and meditation. The common thread running throughout these tales is a sense of disconnection or dissatisfaction with strict religious upbringings.

A JOURNEY FROM DISCONNECTION TO CLARITY

My early years were spent growing up in suburban Australia in the 1970s. As we know, this was a time of cultural change. I was feeling a disturbing disconnection within myself, between what we were taught at school—the importance of education, preparing women for careers, and spirituality—vs. religion, which did not apply to more conservative norms that I was seeing in daily life.

It was in our physical education classes at school that I first encountered yoga. There was something immediately captivating about its direct relationship with the body. The sense of mastery over our physicality made me feel independent. This was my first taste of freedom, a glimpse into a world of relating the external with more self-control.

Yoga has been a constant throughout my life from a young age. Starting with seeing the Beatles in the media with their exotic outfits and Swami Saraswathi on the television with her leopard-print leotards looking glamorous and serene. Something in me was thinking "I want to have what they are having!," which led me to the curiosity and later the passion for Eastern philosophy.

My journey led me to study acupuncture and Eastern philosophy, which at the time was deeply embedded in the training. Mantra and meditation became my anchors, my deep personal connection to yoga. I take this connection seriously, understanding that we all see things according to what's in our mind. This realization is fantastically liberating.

My yoga path has been one of practice, study with teachers, work with professional yoga organizations and teaching. Apart from the connection to a world-wide *sangha*, there are two processes that I feel provided breakthroughs from some of the darker parts of my mind to more sustained lightness and clarity.

A defining moment in my transformation came when I was about 26, attending a residential teacher training in India. The first three weeks were pure misery. I rebelled against every aspect—the early wake-up calls, the food, the sleeping arrangements. We all hated it. They pushed us to our limits, changing our routines, waking us up in the middle of the night to change cabins, making us scrub toilets. It was a classic breaking of the ego.

That discipline broke through a lot of ego-driven silliness. I started to look at how I was holding so strongly to my individual wants and desires, even when they were not making me happy! By the end of the training, I experienced five days of pure bliss. After the weeks of internal struggle, now I didn't want to leave. I would see this as an experience of *karma yoga*—how our actions, the way we live, our perception of our day-to-day can fulfil or disturb us. I never lost that awareness.

After that transformative teacher training, I truly saw how I created my own unhappiness. I remember returning to Australia, sitting on the beach, watching the waves, and feeling a profound sense of timelessness and evenness of mind. I no longer needed to grasp for the next experience or feel that things should be different than they were. It was a blissful experience of just being, with nowhere to go and no one to be.

A decade later I was given the task of preparing Patanjali's *Yoga Sutras* study for a 750-hour teacher training that I was facilitating. Although I had had the privilege of extensive education on the subject, I decided to spend some hours at my desk each day, examining how to teach the essence of each sutra to the yoga teacher trainees.

Through this process I encountered how Patanjali's *Yoga Sutras* provide a concise and practical framework for the human experience. This yoga philosophy course I took sealed the deal for me. Patanjali so eloquently describes how our life is created in our mind, and our ability to direct the course of our mind to clarity. I noticed that the more I immersed myself in the text, the less reactive my mind became. Patanjali reminded me to get out of my own way to allow in the presence.

I was very touched by the way the text is so nonjudgmental and humanitarian. This allowed me a kinder relationship to myself and others. It is within our capacity to create virtuous patterns that give us greater stability and lightness in life. I began to see that experiences come first, and then the science of yoga helps us understand what's happening.

When asked about mystical experiences, I find myself hesitating. Are they so normal that I don't even notice their mystical nature? I often notice synchronicities, sometimes six times in a day. If I'm using psychic capacities, I wouldn't identify them as such—they just feel normal. Our culture doesn't recognize these aspects of ourselves. We're surprised when animals sense things before they happen, like birds flying away before a storm, but we, humans, have similar capabilities. We just don't talk about it, and we have lost that awareness.

For me, yoga is a way of life, an attitude that permeates every aspect of existence. The idea of "yoga on the mat" and everything else being separate doesn't make sense to me. Yoga is about moral conduct and self-discipline. It's about making a yogic decision in every moment, adhering to a particular conduct and way of speaking. In *yoga dharma*, nothing is separate.

The path of yoga is one of nonconformity—trying to think beyond our own conditioned mind and society's expectations. Ironically, the modern yoga movement has become one of the most conformist. In the past, yoga education was about breaking the ego, challenging the need to be accepted, liked, comfortable, or happy. Fundamentally, my experience has been that the less we are concerned with our self-image, the closer we can become to the unchanging, universal principles of yoga.

Certainly, life can always present us with challenges, but the practice of returning to the state of yoga reminds me that there's always an aspect of myself that is awake, aware, and unaffected by any turmoil. The first four of Patanjali's *Yoga Sutras* speak to me, reminding me that we all have the capacity to be fully alive, fully functioning, very healthy, and very present in the moment. We have a choice—we can transform the mind into this clear and present state. This understanding has become the cornerstone of my practice and my teaching, a testament to the transformative power of yoga in my life.

Leanne Davis
C-IAYT, Doctor of Acupuncture, Bachelor of Health Science
(Acupuncture), Yoga Therapist, Vedic Chanting Teacher, Australia

FROM DOGMA TO *DHARMA*: A RABBI'S DAUGHTER'S JOURNEY TO YOGA THERAPY

As a daughter of a rabbi, I was brought up in a very Jewish religious environment with very strict rules. I had a very clear delineation of how my life was supposed to be; my upbringing was full of dogma and doctrine. In our world there's right and there's wrong; there's a way to live and a way not to live. There's a lot of very clear instructions on how to be as a good Jewish woman within the culture.

I always had a sneaking feeling that something was wrong, that I just didn't fit in. For example, we were discouraged from going to college and university for fear that we would get sucked into a secular culture and be influenced by the non-Jewish world. I always valued an education and wanted to become a professional, even though women were discouraged from studying and pursuing careers outside of Jewish education. The consequence of leaving the religion, we were told, would be that we would ultimately be responsible for the destruction of the Jewish nation.

I felt very much this was the reality—we were groomed for marriage and having kids and teaching them about Judaism. That was sort of the pinnacle of our hopes and dreams—how to be a good wife and mother to perpetuate the culture and the Jewish faith. These were my roots and I was committed to my path. I was passionate about it. I did get married at the age of 21 to the perfect Jewish guy.

Then the big shocking event happened—my father, a rabbi, was arrested for dealing drugs—heroin—which was unheard of in our community. This is what I call the crack in the windshield, which is like when all of a sudden you think, this can't even be happening; it's so unreal. Divorce is more normal. Disease is more normal. This was way off the charts. When I asked my father about his crime, he told me he never wanted to see me again, and we didn't speak for 10 years.

This event crushed my construct of the world that I had grown up in. We were shunned by the Jewish community. There was no room for being authentic or real. There were no open emotions. I started to question everything. The life we had led all of a sudden fell apart, and the people who were supposed to be righteous and the most religious were the most disgusting and the most shaming, and the most uncompassionate. That was the initiating event that sort of broke down my reality.

I was 23 and studying Physiotherapy at McGill University at the time, and found solace with my non-Jewish friends who seemed to accept me for who I was. There, I didn't feel shamed by them for the actions of my father.

As I began to open to new people from different cultures, I started to notice that I had been raised to be closed-minded to other people and other cultures. I began to look more for things that made my heart feel good. I started to do things I loved doing but hadn't previously been exposed to—like theater, dance, spending time in nature, surfing, and swimming in the ocean. I needed to feel connected to myself and to something greater.

Then I discovered yoga. I would go in with a storm of thoughts, and after a class I would feel some space between myself and my thoughts. I found my teacher, Aadil Palkhivala, at a conference; he was a lifelong student of BKS Iyengar, but his spiritual teachers were Sri Aurobindo and Mother. He created Purna Yoga and I mostly learned everything about yoga from him.

I was going through a lot of difficulties at that time. I was divorced with a young son. I had been shunned by my community and by my family. But I felt that I was okay, there was a sense that in yoga I'd tapped into something bigger than myself. I had a feeling that I was on the right path. There was a quality of quietness in the souls of all my teachers or in their being, and I really wanted to have a part of that.

Every moment I spent in the yoga studio or studying felt very much like I had tapped into something that was true for everyone and that it didn't matter who you were and what your background was. I felt a deep knowing in my heart that I was exactly where I needed to be, even if my family didn't approve. I had never experienced that before in my life.

I started to realize that yoga also helped me with my own back pain and scoliosis. I realized that I could integrate it into physiotherapy, which was my profession by then. Yoga allowed me to have a relationship with my patients and to see them in a more holistic way than I was taught in the Western model of physiotherapy. I started to insist on seeing people for an hour, which enabled me to be present, to hear them and really see them, which to me was much more rewarding and made more sense. And consequently, my clients did better.

A lot of my yoga studies focused on healing injuries and therapeutic applications. I would say that I came into yoga therapy very much through the physical realm. And then, I added in breathing meditation, the presence, the spirituality. It led me to study somatic psychotherapy so that I could really work much deeper on a soul level with people, helping them find their *dharma* and their purpose in life, letting go of their limiting beliefs and behaviors. That's what I'm interested in now. I found my *dharma* in yoga therapy.

In our yoga therapy school we are giving yoga teachers the gift of going deeper, and understanding the depth that yoga has. We are not prescriptive. We teach core principles that should inform every session. We're teaching people how to relate to other people with love and presence, and we have exercises to teach that. I think that we've come up with a model that emphasizes the principles of yoga therapy, that combines all parts and all styles of yoga. At its heart it's about connecting people to their *dharma* and guiding them to find out who they really are.

Rachel Krentzman
PT, E-RYT, C-IAYT, Physiotherapist, Yoga Therapist,
Author and Hakomi Psychotherapist, Israel

HEALING THROUGH SELF-DISCOVERY

Growing up in a strict Lutheran church, my first spiritual crisis hit me when I was told my three-week-old brother was in hell because he hadn't been baptized. That moment shattered my understanding of God, and set me on a winding path that would span decades.

By 16, I was living a different life entirely. As I entered college, my parents signed affidavits of nonsupport—they couldn't afford my schooling, but their emotional support never wavered. I remember my father driving around just to check if I was okay while I was living in my car and on the road, working as a waitress, dabbling in drugs, and struggling to find my way.

One pivotal moment came during a cocaine run in the mountains. I called my father because I had abandoned my car, and he, guided by his love for me and in his wisdom, arranged a therapy appointment. This led to a Jesus meeting that changed something in me. I could argue the precepts and couldn't argue with the pure love I felt in that room—a total acceptance of who I was, filling an emptiness I hadn't even recognized.

The universe wasn't done with me yet. Shortly after, while changing a flat tire, the car fell on me. I managed to escape, and later, at a restaurant, a man named Buster approached me, saying I had survived because God had a purpose for me to fulfil. His words struck deep, although my journey wasn't over. For the next several years I wrestled with drug use while spending part of the time working with Youth for Christ, trying to help others while still struggling myself.

In my 30s, I discovered yoga at Kripalu. It was there I heard Amrit speak about how people live their lives in boxes—keeping friends and groups with different interests separate, afraid that if anyone knew the whole truth, no one would love them. His words about yoga bringing everything together to make you whole resonated deeply with my fragmented existence.

The dark night of my soul lasted about nine years, through my 30s, 40s, and 50s. It was a time of unlearning, of questioning everything I'd been taught. At around 41, I had a breakdown that became a breakthrough. Standing there, cursing at God, I realized I couldn't return to my old coping mechanisms of scotch, drugs, and needles. Something had fundamentally changed.

Today, my spiritual practice looks different. I wake each morning asking, "What do you want me to do today?" Not expecting booming voices or dramatic signs, but trusting in the quiet guidance that comes through living mindfully. I've learned to live into questions rather than demanding immediate answers. Sometimes my greatest teachers weren't the gurus I sought—like when cancer became my teacher instead.

My journey has profoundly influenced my work as a yoga therapist. I see clients as spirits navigating their own challenges, and I meet them wherever they are—physical, mental, or spiritual. Whether I'm helping someone walk again or guiding them through trauma, it's all about connecting them back to their own source of strength.

The most important lesson I've learned? Trust the unknown. Trust the void. Life rarely shows up the way we expect, and that's exactly as it should be. Through chanting, *pranayama*, and daily practice, I've found that spirituality isn't about dramatic revelations; it's about living moment to moment, breath by breath, in harmony with whatever comes our way.

I was looking for a guru, and I got cancer. And cancer became my guru. I recently just went through a difficult situation with a real estate agent. I lived the question, what am I supposed to be learning from this? And the thing is, I don't need an answer. I think it's more important to live into the answer than worry about it. That's part of spirituality—I don't have to have a reason for everything. I can just be with it, and life will take care of itself. This way I feel that I'm living my *dharma*.

If something's not working quite right, I hold the question and say—is this to find my perseverance and resilience, because this is where I need to go? Or is this a red flag to step away and follow a different direction? Then I open myself up for the answer. It's living moment to moment without having to have an expectation of how it's going to show up.

Looking back at that lost young woman living an unfocused, lost, purposeless but searching life, I wish I could tell her that all those struggles were leading somewhere meaningful. That one day, she'd help others find their way back to wholeness—not despite her broken path, but because of it.

Hansa Knox
C-IAYT, E-RYT-500, YACEP, owner of PranaYoga and Āyurveda Mandala, Yoga & Yoga Therapy School and Studio, USA

FROM CATHOLIC TO SWAMI: A JOURNEY THROUGH YOGA AND SELF-DISCOVERY

I was locking my bike up outside a health food store in New York City one day and somehow ended up in a yoga class next door. It was an awkward experience, but after the class I was struck by an unexplainable new awareness. A seed was planted. Life put me on a spiritual journey. I had grown up Catholic and tried to make it work, even through college, but ended up putting it aside.

At 30, I moved to Los Angeles. My personal life became extremely challenging. I started clenching my teeth, even broke a tooth. I needed help. I heard they served food after the classes at Sivananda Yoga. That sounded welcoming. I went to a trial class. The teacher said, "Lie down on the mat and relax." I remember warm tears escaping from my eyes in *shavasana*. Permission to let go. I started going to yoga. Every day. My car ended up at the yoga center even if I was intending to go elsewhere. I practiced *asana* and *pranayama* regularly for *years*.

Having become a "regular," I thought I should check out Sunday evening *satsang*. My eyes were open for all 30 minutes of the silent meditation. I stumbled through the chants. Then the swami fielded questions I didn't even know you could ask. Wow. There was a lightness in my step as I walked back to my car. I felt *happier*. I never missed a Sunday after that. I gradually learned to empty my mind and fill it with higher thinking.

Then I summoned the courage to try a *puja*, not really knowing what it was. It was Swami Sivananda's birthday. There was only the swami, one staff member...and me. They encouraged me to stay, sat me down with a big bowl of red rose petals in front of the most beautiful picture of Swami Sivananda, and said, "Just offer the flower petals." His kind eyes were so alive, so deep. I was overwhelmed by the love! My heart cracked open.

I felt more fit and was eating better, breathing better, and feeling my feelings. I was able to relax. I had a new "family" who accepted me exactly as I was. I will never forget the staff and regular students who were supporting the center at that time!

One day, in the reception area, they were announcing an upcoming trip to South India planned by the international Sivananda Yoga organization. Out of my mouth came, "Sign me up!" I looked over my shoulder. Who said that? I felt unprepared, but impelled to go. In India, my heart *burst* open.

Maybe it wasn't a near-death experience, but after our day visiting the temple in Rameshwaram toward the end of the pilgrimage, I was not the same. I woke up in the middle of the night. Apparently, it was hot, but I was *freezing cold*. I remember touching my face, which felt smooth, like porcelain, and asking, "Who am I? Was that my life?" I felt peaceful; there was no fear. In the morning, I knew I had been through a very deep purification.

At 36, I completed the Sivananda Yoga Teacher Training Course—for my own personal practice, or so I thought. Right away, I started to teach and never stopped. Something was coming through me. The results were out of my hands. I experienced surrender. *Karma* yoga (selfless service) became a joy. I didn't want to miss any opportunity to serve this mission of Peace.

I had set up an altar at home. I got up at 5.30am daily to meditate, chant, and read on my own. It became a habit for life. I love to demystify meditation for students. It is all about the mind detaching.

The teachings of *Vedanta* dawned. Perspective continued to shift. I am not this body or this mind. I am not a New Yorker. I am not an Angeleno. I am not my job. I am not my house. I am not my talents. I am not my shortcomings. What is this freedom?

At 53, I had decided to spend one month per year at the most peaceful place I knew—the Sivananda Yoga Farm in Grass Valley, California. But instead, I moved in! I don't think I had been there three months when Swami Sitaramananda suggested, "I think you should be the director of the new San Francisco center." I was cringing inside, "No, I just got here…" But outside, I heard myself saying, "Yes, Swamiji!" She asked, "Could you give 10 years to the San Francisco center?" The same voice that had taken me to India calmly said, "Yes."

In a corner of the new center we had just purchased, we noticed termites. When the exterminator came, he announced, "Lady, termites are the least of your problems; there's water inside the wall." I shocked myself with the calm thought, "I wonder how *that's* going to work out?" Of course, it's going to. What a relief from my old thinking!

I saw, over and over, that things simply worked out. The surrender, the purification, was unfolding.

As director, I would make a report of our weekly income every Sunday. I started to notice something uncanny. The total income always seemed *less* than the total expenditure, and yet, over time, the money in the bank remained steady. Divine economics? I learned not to question.

Another time, the ashram priest arrived with a beautiful white marble Siva lingam. It had been carved in Vietnam for the San Francisco center. "It should sit on a brass plate," he instructed. I grabbed a tape measure. Fourteen inches should do it. We searched online and in the local Indian stores, but could not find a 14-inch brass plate. A few weeks later, my brother called. "Mom and I were going through a cabinet in her dining room and found a 14-inch brass plate from India—could you use it?"

I also became a yoga therapist, synthesizing all the tools of yoga in service of perfect health—truly a rich "lifestyle medicine."

I was 57 when I took vows and became a swami, dedicating my life to the highest realization of yoga or Oneness. I wear orange to remind me.

There were so many lessons I needed to learn—and repeat—to get to this point. I am grateful for those experiences, hard as they were, that helped me break through my fantasies, face my ego, and see myself, my True Self. What I was seeking was not outside. Everything is inside. The joy is inside. That freedom, that joy, is the source of all healing!

Swami Sivasankariananda
Director, Los Angeles Sivananda Yoga Vedanta Center, USA

JOURNEY OF SPIRITUAL TRANSFORMATION

I grew up in a house divided. My mother, a fervent evangelical Christian, wielded religion like a sword, while my father, a Deist and abstract mathematician, approached life with a more open-minded curiosity. This stark contrast left me feeling torn and confused, especially when my mother's harsh words about eternal damnation cut deep into my young heart.

"You're going to hell if you don't accept Jesus as your personal Savior," my mother would say, leaving me feeling hollow and worthless.

Despite the suffocating atmosphere at home, I always felt a connection to something greater. My dreams often seemed prophetic, offering glimpses into future events with uncanny accuracy. One night, at the tender age of 11, I experienced a vivid encounter that would shape my destiny.

In my dream, I found myself awake in my bedroom, aware that I was dreaming, yet unable to move. A presence materialized in the corner—a figure with dreadlocks, emanating an aroma of camphor and incense.

As I entered my teenage years, the weight of my conflicted upbringing and spiritual confusion plunged me into a deep depression. At my lowest point, I attempted to take my own life, believing there was no escape from the darkness that engulfed me.

Years passed, and I found myself trapped in a cycle of work and exhaustion. At 37, I was burning the candle at both ends, working impossibly long hours and traveling constantly. It was during this time that a chance encounter with a yoga class advertisement caught my eye.

"Why not?" I thought, seeking nothing more than a bit of exercise.

Little did I know that this simple decision would change the course of my life. As I lay on my mat during the final relaxation, tears streamed down my face. For the first time in years, I felt a profound sense of peace and calm. It was as if a long-locked door had finally creaked open, allowing a sliver of light to penetrate the darkness.

Determined to hold on to this newfound serenity, I sought out teachers who could guide me deeper into the practice. I found Laura and Bhava, whose Deep Yoga school became my sanctuary. Under their guidance, I began to peel away the layers of pain and self-doubt that had accumulated over the years.

Laura, a yoga therapist and Ayurvedic practitioner, became my weekly confidante. She introduced me to *japa mala mantra* and prescribed a nourishing diet of kitchari as I let go of my dependence on alcohol and cigarettes. Slowly, but surely, the walls I had built to protect myself began to crumble, revealing the authentic self I had long forgotten.

During my yoga teacher training, I accepted a challenge that would prove transformative: waking up between 4 and 6am each day to practice. At first, I could barely manage to stay in child's pose for 20 minutes, often dissolving into tears. But as the days turned into weeks, and weeks into months, something miraculous happened—the cloud of depression that had followed me for so long disappeared, to never come back.

"Make your own definition of spirituality," my teacher had said. "You can call it the light, the energy of the universe, whatever resonates with you."

These words were a balm to my soul, soothing the wounds left by years of rigid religious doctrine. I began to explore my own understanding of spirituality, free from the fear and judgment that had haunted my childhood.

As I deepened my practice, I found myself better equipped to handle life's challenges. When my parents fell ill—my mother injured in an accident and my father battling Parkinson's disease—I drew upon the strength I had cultivated through yoga. The *durga mantra* became my constant companion, carrying me through the difficult tasks of caregiving and managing my parents' affairs.

Today, I stand as a beacon of hope for others struggling to find their path. As a yoga teacher, I dedicate my classes to joy and self-transformation, always ending with the deeply restorative practice of *yoga nidra*. I honor the roots of yoga while making the practice accessible to students from all walks of life and spiritual backgrounds.

"I'm not here to tell you what to believe," I often tell my diverse group of students near the Mexican border. "I'm here to offer you tools that can support you on your own spiritual journey, wherever it may lead."

My journey from a confused and depressed young woman to a compassionate and grounded yoga teacher is a testament to the transformative power of self-discovery. By embracing my own unique spirituality and letting go of the need to conform to others' expectations, I found the peace and purpose that had eluded me for so long.

As I guide my students to connect with their own hearts, I know that the real healing happens when we create space for others to find their own truth. My story serves as a reminder that even in our darkest moments, a spark of light remains—waiting for us to fan it into a flame of self-realization and inner peace.

Kari Ross-Berry
E-RYT-500, YACEP, C-IAYT, Associate Professor of Exercise Science:
Yoga at Southwestern College, Lead Teacher: Yoga Therapy Rx at Loyola
Marymount University, MA in Yoga Studies, MS in Exercise Science, USA

FROM CATHOLIC ROOTS TO YOGIC WINGS

I was adopted and raised in a devout Catholic family on the East Coast, with my mother especially committed to Catholicism. I vividly remember sitting in church, feeling a pull toward something deeper. I would think to myself, "When I grow up, I'm going to bring all religions together and create a church of my own." It was only later I discovered that such thoughts were considered unconventional, but this early sense of spiritual curiosity stayed with me, pushing me to look beyond organized religion.

Growing up, I felt different as an adopted child, and my parents were protective, sometimes even insecure about my knowledge of my biological family. Despite this complex emotional landscape, I found solace in yoga, even before

I knew what it was. For as long as I could remember, I was doing headstands and sitting in *sukhasana*. I also tried to teach myself meditation, seeking a sense of peace.

After college, I moved to California. I was looking for a job and made my way into a small music store, where I found work as a piano teacher. Shortly after, the owner discovered I had a background in business and asked me to manage the store. It wasn't a high-paying role, but they offered something far more valuable to me—an opportunity to learn yoga and meditation in exchange for my work.

In a synchronistic turn, I met my future husband through the music store. His mother had been a devotee of Yogananda, and from the moment we met, I felt a profound connection. We've been married for many decades and have four adult children together.

In the 1990s, I discovered Deepak Chopra's teachings, which resonated with me by integrating both philosophy and science. Attending a meditation retreat at the Chopra Center was a turning point. For a week, I immersed myself in all things yoga. Through the center, I earned meditation, yoga *asana*, and Ayurveda certifications.

Over the years, my career shifted from music to writing, and I worked for a long time in speechwriting and media relations. Not long after a silent retreat with the center, where I set an intention to focus solely on writing about yoga and its many modalities, I received a call to write several of Deepak's 21-day meditation programs, and helped grow the audience by thousands of listeners.

I was also invited to lead meditation workshops, drawing large groups eager to explore yogic teachings. Eventually, I left my other freelance work to focus entirely on writing and teaching on yogic topics. I also helped develop online courses on meditation and Ayurveda for the Chopra Center, and taught for many years as a member of the center's lead faculty.

In recent years, I graduated from the MA in Yoga program at Loyola Marymount University, where I discovered yoga therapy. That program, and its postgraduate Yoga Therapy certificate, felt like a culmination of everything I had been moving toward. Whether through writing or direct practice, I sensed yoga therapy was the work I was meant to do—helping others align with their inner voice.

Throughout my journey, I've relied on guidance that I've felt somatically and intuitively. Now, I see my life as a continuous journey of spiritual evolution. Each step, even if it has appeared unconventional from the outside, has brought me closer to alignment. A teacher once told me that intuition is always right, although not everyone is attuned to hear it. I believe yoga therapy holds the potential to guide people back to that inner voice, helping them align and listen to their own guidance.

Susan Chapman®
MA, MFA, PGYT, C-IAYT, E-RYT 500, YTRx™-1000, POLY, YACEP, Yoga Therapist, Instructor, Scholar, and Coach, USA

CHAPTER 8

The Gift of Yoga

The following six stories weave together themes of personal transformation, unexpected encounters with the divine, and the powerful gift of yoga to bridge the gap between the physical and spiritual realms.

TRANSFORMATIVE ENCOUNTERS: A JOURNEY FROM SOLDIER TO YOGA THERAPIST

I came to yoga by accident. I wasn't looking for spirituality. It happened this way. I served in the Australian Army during the Vietnam War and was sent to Papua New Guinea. I became drawn to the local culture, visited tribal villages, and I attended some ceremonies. It opened me up to seeing things in a different way and not through the rational lens I'd learned in college. This laid the groundwork for what was yet to come.

Back in Australia a few years later, I went to yoga class. It was an *Iyengar* class and it kicked my butt. I talked to a friend who had spent some time with Sai Baba. He told me about a whole different world of yoga. So, I began to attend practices at the Satyananda Yoga Ashram in the Adelaide Hills. One of the senior swamis came for a lecture in the college where I was teaching. He asked me if he could teach yoga in the college and I helped him to make it happen. I was also doing practices at home. My eldest daughter—eight at the time—came to me and said, "Dad, I like when you do yoga because you are not so grumpy afterwards." And she was right and I could sense that.

My college teaching focus was administrative behavior and was focused on personal and organizational change—how do we change our behavior? I would lead workshops on the topic, and although the participants would leave inspired, nothing much would change in their behavior. After a while I understood that there was no change in behavior because the learning was all cognitive. The workshops were not experiential like my yoga practice, and it was in the practice, and the experiential awareness that came with it, that the power to change resided.

I realized I needed an expanded experience of yoga. With my next sabbatical, I decided to go and live in an ashram and chose Kripalu (which was then an ashram) in the Northeast USA. For a year I studied the impact of yoga and meditation on myself experientially, as part of my dissertation for a Master's degree. It was 1984 when I wrote my thesis on the transformational power of yoga therapy, supervised by faculty from a college in Vermont.

During that time, I had many metaphysical experiences. One was when I was holding triangle pose for an extended time. We were playing at the time with the idea of *pratyahara*. Can you go from external awareness to internal experience? My mentor, the late Don Stapleton, was helping me to hold triangle pose, and I was at the point of quitting and changing it to another posture. In that moment he put his hand on my heart and said—take another breath. I took the breath and then I just felt I dropped in—*bang*! I was in different state. I don't know how long I stayed there, and I could have stayed there forever it was so beautiful.

This experience was very revealing, and I am told that it was very similar to an experience with psychedelics. I was, however, in a different state of consciousness—it was reality where everything was okay, nothing to fear. It revealed to me my own fears. I had a flashback to when I was small boy, about eight years old, in the school playground, being beaten by bigger boys. And I felt the terror of that moment. That was a huge release.

After I came out, I noticed I was quite ungrounded. During that experience I had images and sensory experiences, but I didn't formulate the story connected to experience. I only got to the story when I went back to my room afterwards and started to journal. The experience itself wasn't cognitive; it was physical, emotional, and spiritual. It was a felt sense without much figuring out or mental processing.

Another experience I had was in a room of about 200 people practicing daily *sadhana*. I could really feel the collective energy when we practiced together. On that particular day I was in camel pose and I could feel my whole body open and feel like it was completely hollow. I couldn't distinguish the boundaries between my body and the air around me. It was all one. It was scary at first, and then it felt beautiful. I was able to embrace the vulnerability, and in that I found my strength. And when I brought this attitude to life—that became really powerful.

By the time I finished my thesis and left the ashram I wanted to engage in yoga therapy professionally. I went back to Australia and resigned from a fully tenured professorship at the college and returned to the USA and Kripalu to practice yoga therapy.

More and more I took refuge on my yoga mat in my *sadhana*, particularly in times of vulnerability. At the beginning of my practice, I could notice and feel the vulnerability, but find strength growing from the inside as I continued with my practice. I related this to a friend who said it reminded him of the story of the phoenix rising from the ashes. The name Phoenix Rising came to me, and was to be the name of my work going forward.

To this day, decades later, the experiential understanding of yoga remains the focus of my work. This internal aspect of yoga is indeed spiritual. But it doesn't matter where the people are coming from to practice yoga. You don't have to own or sprout spirituality to get to it. Any place is a good place to start, and eventually, with consistent practice—*sadhana*—you will find Spirit in yoga.

It is still important for me to engage my own practice. People say to me, "Ah you are old, you've done this for 40 years—you've made it." My answer to this is—*no*! I still need to learn, to do my own work, and to continue to transform so I can better serve others. I need my own *sadhana*. I still practice daily and go to meditation retreats whenever the opportunity comes.

Michael Lee
MA, DipSocSci, C-IAYT, Founder of Phoenix Rising Yoga Therapy, USA

TOUCHING THE CENTER

Early in my yoga practice I began having mystical or psychic experiences resulting from, I believe, my meditation practice. These showings have continued throughout my life of yoga, in minor forms, but these were the beginnings and most potent realities. I never looked for or craved any of this. In fact, I was a bit nervous about what was happening to me. I knew from the master's teachings and warnings (Sri Swami Satchidananda)—there was no credit given, no encouragement for seeking or craving higher consciousness.

"Worry about OSP [ordinary sensory perception] not ESP [extrasensory perception]," Swamiji would always chide. "How you close the door, how you greet your neighbor" mattered more, we were always warned.

Hence, if you had any of these things happening, and you were a shy and quiet introvert, as I was, you said nothing to anyone. So it was worrying. These experiences were not invited, only endured.

They began with astral travel. My guess is because I was so at home at the yoga center at night when I went to sleep part of me would fly back to be there in this space. This experience would sometimes frighten me—flapping through the dark and breezy night sky and down through the rumbling subway tunnel, my usual route to Greenwich Village from my home apartment near Yankee Stadium on 161st Street in the Bronx was the path my "spirit" would travel to get to the Integral Yoga Institute (the IYI) in Greenwich Village. Intuitively, within time, I learned to stay grounded in my body, and then these happenings subsided. After that I would have visions of saintly ochre-clad swamis seated in cross-legged positions levitating over my bed, as if guarding over me. These apparitions were more calming, more reassuring. Within time, they, too, subsided.

Although I said nothing to anyone about this, I did know from reading yoga books that these occurrences could happen. My life was simple, quiet, and deeply interior. Aside from schoolwork, there was volunteer work at the yoga center and casual conversations with other volunteer yogis there, and there was home. I lived alone.

Overall, I felt secure, protected in this uncanniness. I never feared that anything bad or negative was happening to me. I believed in God, a benevolent universe, and the law of *karma*, and tried to honor this in life. I never felt the grips of sin or the devil (as some folks, usually Christian students of mine, would later surmise about) at any time during these happenings as a young 24-year-old New York University (NYU) college student.

I was a sincere seeker and student of yoga who sat regularly for meditation, particularly in the morning—same time, same place, same ritual. On many occasions I went to the IYI on 13th Street in Manhattan to meditate, but then there were other times during school breaks or when the weather was bad, particularly in the winter months, when I would meditate at home. In any case, this was one of those occasions where I got up in the morning and sat on my meditation cushion in front of my little altar at home and began my morning ritual.

Usually, after an opening prayer, I did some breathing practices to steady my mind, and then I would sit in silent meditation. This particular morning started exactly like all the others; the only thing is, once I completed my breathing practice and began repeating the mantra, within what seemed like minutes I sank into a deep meditative state. I don't know what else happened; all I do know is that I then opened my eyes after what seemed like just a few minutes. I had all intentions of settling back into my meditation again, because in my mind I had just started and had barely been meditating for more than 5 or 10 minutes. Then I just happened to glance at my clock and saw that two hours had passed—what felt to me like two minutes! I could not believe that this was so. I was sure there was something amiss with my clock.

I got up and walked into the kitchen to check the clock there. It showed the same time. I was bemused. This had never happened before. I had had times of quiet meditation, but never had I lost consciousness of time like this! Another thing I noticed after this meditation was that I was totally at ease, at peace—with myself, and with my world. "This feels different," I thought, as I bathed and dressed and proceeded to leave the house. I still had not comprehended what I had experienced.

Every moment was a new revelation. As soon as I stepped outside the door of my apartment building into the new day, everything felt different…the air, the sounds, the light. The physical world did not seem the same. In fact, I felt that although I was able to navigate my physical environment, I was clearly far removed from it. This separation was very real to me, and what was more startling was the fact that I no longer felt affected by the world! I was at peace with everything! I was at peace with the class that I was struggling with at university, I was at peace with so-called friends who found me too freaky-calm these days, I was at peace with being a financially poor college student in an upper-middle-class student body environment. I was at peace with spending much time alone, at peace with my appearance, at peace with the weather, the time of day, the day of the week. I was at peace with strangers, with the rich and poor alike. I was at peace with those who looked happy and those who looked sad, I was at peace with myself and with my God. This consciousness I felt shielded and protected me. I feared nothing, not even death!

This heightened consciousness remained with me for at least a few days or maybe weeks, I am not quite sure anymore. All I do know is that slowly, over time, it subsided. Fear returned. Restlessness returned. The only thing that did not return was my doubt about the existence of something out there greater, bigger than me, than us, which was invariably in control. This was undeniable for me now. I could not undo this loss of ignorance!

Joanne Wohlmuth
MA, E-RYT-500, YACEP, C-IAYT, Yoga Trainer/Instructor/
OD Consultant at Yoga On The Rock, Bermuda

WEAVING SCIENCE AND SPIRITUALITY: A JOURNEY OF INQUIRY AND CONNECTION

I was born into a Jewish family. When I was 12 and preparing to become a Bat Mitzvah, I told my rabbi that I was agnostic, that I wasn't sure if I believed in G-d. Her response was so important for the future of my Jewish identity and my spiritual journey. She said, "It's very Jewish to question." She explained that intellectual inquiry and spiritual inquiry were a rich part of Jewish tradition. It gave me permission to be uncertain, and placed value on the process of inquiry as part of a rich cultural tradition.

Many years later, I have a career as a research scientist. It is my job to question. In science, as in spirituality, every question brings another question. In the scientific process and in spirituality, there are different ways of seeing, perceiving, and understanding. I have had experiences that led me to question what I know is true. At this point in my journey, my uncertainty is not about whether there is a concept of divinity, but what that actually means. Over the years, I have had many experiences that might be characterized as otherworldly. Some of it is very concrete, like a message that seems clear as day. Other times, it is just a felt sense or a kind of intuition.

My first experience of this was during graduate school when I had a summer off and was apartment sitting for a professor. I had no formal responsibilities while school was in recess, and it was one of the most carefree times of my adult life. I meditated every day, practiced yoga, went running outside, prepared fresh meals, read books, watered plants, and drank herbal tea on the balcony. I didn't have a television and it was before smartphones, so I was in almost a constant state of mindfulness with plenty of nourishment and rest. These were probably the most ideal conditions for noticing what is beyond the immediate senses.

I was sitting quietly on the sofa and I started to feel the presence of beings in the room. It happened on a few occasions and included people I knew, like my deceased grandfathers and uncles, but also people I didn't know, like someone I perceived to be an Indigenous elder. I considered the possibility that I might be delusional or conjuring such perceptions, but that just didn't ring true.

Years later, when my daughter was a baby, I could feel the presence of my grandfather, who she was named after. I could tell where he was in the room by the awareness of his presence as I rocked her to sleep.

Since then, I have been periodically sensing messages from departed loved ones that seem to be confirmed when I pass them along. In one instance, my grandmother, who was an incredibly kind-hearted soul, uncharacteristically gave me a message that said, "Pull yourself together!" I somehow knew this was for my father, and when I passed it along, he confirmed that he had been feeling sorry for himself that day and had the thought that his mother would not be proud of his wallowing.

In another instance, I felt my dead mother telling me to literally smell the roses. I didn't realize that on that very day the rose garden at her house had its first bloom of the season.

I don't doubt this anymore, but I don't understand it either. I don't know what G-d means, and I don't know how this all happens. But I do notice all kinds of serendipities because I know that there are realities we will never truly understand. Whether it is my own intuition, the deep knowing of loved ones that lives within me, or actual messages coming from the other side, I feel guided by something that isn't my intellectual mind.

As many traditions teach, we are spiritual beings, and spirituality is part of our personhood. It is part of the *panchamaya kosha* model of yoga and the biopsychosocial-spiritual model of modern science. When I am conducting an intake with a new client as a yoga therapist or as a health coach, I always ask questions about spirituality. Whether the client feels connected to a specific tradition or not, I want to know where their sense of connection comes from. It might be through service to humanity, oneness with the natural world, prayer, or song. What is their unique worldview, and how can I offer practices that will help foster a sense of meaning and purpose beyond the balance of physical health? When we shy away from these questions, it is a disservice to the client and their wholeness.

When we are not taking care of our bodies, when we are not emotionally attuned and aware, when we are not living ethically and morally, it can be more challenging to connect with our spirituality. But that doesn't mean it isn't there, waiting for us to notice. Yoga practices and general self-care have helped me to maintain a greater awareness of spiritual connection, even amidst the challenges of daily life.

It has taken a long time for me to weave together my spiritual path and my religious tradition. It has required that I find my own personal relationship to Jewish ritual and its meaning. For some clients, a sense of spiritual meaning is already alive within their religious practice. For others, their spirituality exists completely outside of any formal tradition. Still others weave the two together in ways that resonate with them. I do not ignore the opportunity for connectedness with something, whatever form that might take.

For those who are scientifically minded, I think there is often a misunderstanding that science is only about measuring what is certain and objectively true. But science is so much more complex than that. Science is about pushing the boundaries of what we understand, and reaching for the next answerable question. At a certain point, we start getting to questions that are unanswerable with our current methodology. But many phenomena that were once beyond the realm of science can now be measured. The line between science and spirituality is a fluid one, and they are not mutually exclusive. In fact, the incredible discoveries that scientists make when exploring the natural world can awaken a powerful sense of awe and wonder. Science itself, therefore, might even be a form of spiritual practice.

Steffany Moonaz
PhD, C-IAYT, Professor and Research Director at Southern California University of Health Sciences, Founder/Director of Yoga for Arthritis, USA

SADHANA AND SELF-DISCOVERY

I don't know when I might have realized that I am aware of being a spiritual being and aware of something more, something bigger than me. Something that is powerful, universal, guiding, caring, supporting all of that. I think I came in to this incarnation remembering and knowing that.

I picked a preacher and a teacher for my parents. They were guides and teachers that were going to allow me to blossom in a safe space during a time when there was not a safe space in the whole country for a Black person. What you see is a presentation of a Black woman. But this is not my ultimate identity. My mom sung us awake each morning. My dad was an army chaplain. We didn't wake up with fear of who we were as Black people.

I attribute that to their spirituality and their faith. I remember when I was a kid, I was deathly afraid of death. It was daily in my thoughts and in a daily prayer. I remember this guidance from my dad, which I thought was such good news.

He said "Don't worry about this whole idea of heaven and hell. Just do what you know is right in your heart. God is in you. God loves you, just do what God guides you to do. Don't do it because you're trying to get to heaven."

"Well, but Dad, how do we get to heaven?"

"You know, maybe there's a heaven. Maybe there's no heaven."

"But I don't want to go to hell."

"Yeah, maybe there's no hell. You do what God puts on your heart to do."

This stuck with me and I think, I got this freedom to explore with the knowing that I am loved and that I'm held. And then this miracle happens...

My child had a severe asthma attack. She was in hospital in ICU for days and I was sleeping with her. The nurse came to me and patted me on my hand and said: "We've done everything we could and we will just have to wait to see what happens."

I called my mom and told her that. And then 15 minutes later my parents, who lived in another city, appeared in the room, like, fell from the sky into the room. I was surprised and asked them: "How come you could so quickly come here??!!"

"You need our support. You need all of our energetic support, too, because we got to get your child back."

Ten days later we got my daughter in a good place. One of the things that I learned is, you're not on this journey by yourself—you have angels all along the way. The other angel in that experience was a doctor who had been doing research on asthma medications. He said that the meds my daughter was given had an ingredient to which she was very allergic—so he gave us some tips to help her. We wanted Grace to become his patient but he said he was just a researcher and left. We were trying to find him somehow but we didn't even know his name! The miracles are the things unexplained. I live them every day, I see them every day...

I started out hot yoga and loved it. I needed a stress release. I decided to become a teacher, and I loved the teacher training. And then I kept looking for some more. I took a 300-hour yoga therapist training. And my interest kept me going and looking for more.

I ended up meeting my mentor before I got into the yoga therapy program. Gurgeet needed teachers for the study he was doing, and I got involved. He opened a yoga therapy program and I signed up. Gurgeet told me, "You are not spiritually questing because you already know. Go, be spiritually curious, have fun. But you know who you are." I liked that KYM (Krishnamacharya Yoga Mandiram) didn't interpret too much and just let me download the knowledge and make my own interpretation, be on my own journey. I also learned Vedic chanting and became a teacher of it, too.

I had this stabbing pain in my head. After the first practice with Gurgeet, the pain, for the first time, dissolved! So he gave me some movement and *pranayama* with extended exhale. That became my practice. When I open my eyes at the end of each practice I see these circles, and they are yellow with a light-blue halo. They'll come into clear, crisp focus, or they'll fall and phase away. And usually,

I would have a conversation with my ex-husband's mother. When she passed, I knew because she came to me, in the form of a vision of her head and my head and my husband's head all morphed together. She asked me to look out for him.

How do I know when the guidance comes that it's not my ego? That gets honed with the *sadhana* and the study. Then you know that you know, even if you do not know how you know—it's right in my heart. You do *sadhana* for your own development, not for the self-care.

Without *sadhana* there would be confusion between "Am I doing this?" or "Am I guided?" That confusion is stressful because it creates doubt, fear, "Am I good enough?!" But when you practice you relinquish all that because it's not you. The journey of practice really does help you navigate this life. I believe in daily practice. I think daily practice is the way. And it's non-negotiable.

I went through a journey with my *sadhana*. I used to treat it like a tick-box. And then I went through the whole gaspiness of it. Get out of my way if you're going to mess with my *sadhana*! And then eventually you get into a space where everything actually is opening up to be able to maintain this connection. Of course, I could not have this knowing, this guidance, without *sadhana*. I think they go hand in hand for me in my experience.

I want to be realistic; I don't want anyone to think that you're on this journey to reach perfection. There is no perfection. Every time I think I am done with an issue, *wham*! Something happens and shows me another layer. The deeper I dig, the more stuff comes up! It's a never-ending journey of self-discovery!

Janet M. Caldwell
MS, C-IAYT, Healing Therapist, USA

FROM LUTHERAN ROOTS TO HUMANISTIC SPIRITUALITY THROUGH YOGA

I've never really thought of myself as "on" a spiritual journey—spirituality has been as natural to me as breathing. It's like asking a fish about water; it's always been there, an intrinsic part of my life. My father was a Lutheran minister and we lived in an urban missionary setting, sharing a communal house with other families. Our days revolved around prayer, connection, and service, almost like growing up in a modern-day ashram. Spirituality wasn't something I chose; it was the fabric of my existence.

Even as a child, I was drawn to spiritual questions. When I was just nine years old, I drew a picture and wrote a story—one I still have today—about going to India and meeting a snake. The snake shared all its knowledge with me, which I then brought back to the US. Looking back, it feels like a premonition of the path I was destined to walk. By the time I was eight, I had already begun to explore spiritual paths outside of Lutheranism, asking my father to read to me about Buddhism and other religions. Mysticism fascinated me. I wondered: Who is God? Why are we here? I even wrote a children's book about a little girl trying to figure out what God was. The presence of God was always there, woven into the fabric of my everyday life.

In my 30s, I traveled to India, just as I had imagined as a child, and studied at the Krishnamacharya Yoga Mandiram. It was there I had a moment of clarity: Yoga therapy would be both my spiritual path and my profession. Yoga wasn't just a set of postures; it was a holistic way of life, offering guidance on how to wake up, eat, rest, and live with purpose. For the first time, while in the ashram, I experienced *sattva* for days at a time—that feeling of spaciousness and lightness, where I felt truly connected to something beyond myself.

Regulating my nervous system through yoga has been the greatest spiritual gift. The practice—whether through *asana*, *pranayama*, meditation, chanting, or lifestyle choices—has allowed me to bring myself into balance, body, and mind, so I can better connect to what feels divine. It's not just self-care; it's a non-negotiable daily *sadhana*. For me, it's as essential as breathing. My husband and I often say, "Thank God for yoga therapy," because we truly wouldn't have survived life's stresses and hardships without it.

Without yoga I would likely be on medication and struggling with chaotic relationships. It has brought clarity, helping me avoid getting caught up in drama and confusion. My purpose is clear—teaching yoga, caring for my family, and helping lost animals. These are the three things I want to devote my life to. Without yoga, I doubt I'd be able to give back to my community in the same way.

As I've grown older, my connection to the divine has continued to evolve. In my younger years, I saw it as a more of an internal and external presence. Now, I am beginning to see it in a more humanistic light, one that I like to call humanistic spirituality. It's the idea that our connection to the divine is inseparable from our connection to humanity itself. Humanistic spirituality focuses on compassion, empathy, and kindness—seeing the divine in every person, in every interaction. It's about living a life of purpose—not just for oneself, but for the good of others. It's about recognizing that the sacred is not just something to be found in temples or scriptures, but in our daily lives, in the way we treat others, in the love we show, and the community we build.

For me, humanistic spirituality means that every act of care, every moment of empathy, and every connection with another being is sacred. It's seeing the divine in the eyes of a lost animal, in the warmth of my family, and in the shared breath of a yoga class. It's about finding meaning not just in personal enlightenment, but in how we uplift others in our community.

At the end of the day, when I close my eyes, breathe inward, and quiet my mind, I feel warmth in my heart—a sense of connection. Maybe that's God within. I don't always know for sure, but in those moments of stillness, I trust that I'm tapping into something greater than myself.

Amy Wheeler
PhD, C-IAYT, Optimal State Yoga Therapy School, USA

FROM VISIONS TO YOGA: A LIFE GUIDED BY THE UNSEEN

My mother was a Quaker. My father was an American Baptist minister and later director of the American Youth Foundation in St. Louis, Missouri, where he ran camps for youth. The programs in these camps were designed to bring the spiritual, social, mental, and physical parts of our body together. I attended these camps for 10 years and found the experience to be a very transformative time in my life.

There are two significant events that helped form who I am today. I must have been 14 when I had a dream, and I saw the camp burn. I can remember in my dream standing on a hill and looking down at the cabins as about 10 or 12 cabins completely burned down. So come the last day of camp that summer, a camper's father, not aware, drops a cigarette, causing many of the cabins to burn. It was exactly as I had seen it in my dream several months earlier, and I realized that there is more in life than meets the eye.

The other event happened when I was married with two young children. I was driving to work and had a vision—I saw myself at my husband's funeral, and then I saw myself with my children on a beach, with the blackest, finest sand ever, and we were okay. That very day of my vision my husband was killed in a car accident. A number of years later, friends invited my family to join them with their children to visit their family in Kenya. While there we went to Mombasa. We stayed at this lovely center, and when I opened the gate to go out to the beach, I saw the blackest, prettiest sand ever, and realized my children and I were fine.

Those experiences convinced me that there's a bigger force at play. It connects us all, takes care of us, and also challenges us. Organized religion doesn't speak to me at this time in my life. Yoga and being in nature help me to connect to something bigger in life. My dream and vision were my big "aha" moments… then there are the everyday little ones, like seeing a beautiful tree turn colors, someone's smile, or to witness an act of kindness. These moments are what feeds me spiritually.

I started yoga at a YMCA in my 20s, doing *asanas*. I did this until about 15 years ago when I left administration at a university where I had been a dean for 12 years. During my academic life I have done all kinds of research on family caregiving. On a sabbatical following my administrative role, I read an article about a group in California who were using yoga with family caregivers. I went there for several days just to watch and learn from them, so I might bring it into my research. Yoga helped me relax and calm me down, and I realized that is exactly what caregivers needed. This led to my becoming a member of the International Association of Yoga Therapists.

Also I began yoga training with Amy Weintraub. Locally I started sharing my limited yoga knowledge at the Center of Torture and War Trauma with some Bosnian women. This experience made me seek out a 200-hour yoga teacher program. Several of us in teacher training worked with Bosnian men who had been in concentration camps. I realized that 200 hours of yoga teacher training was still not enough for me, so I enrolled in a 500-hour yoga teacher training. I have used this knowledge to share yoga in several research studies with people who have Alzheimer's disease and women with breast cancer. In bringing yoga to people I often see these big "aha" moments happening. You see people making connections with themselves, their body, and with others. It's a huge gift and honor to me personally, to be part of those moments.

Sometimes I feel led by something bigger than myself, and sometimes I have not known that I was being led, and then, all of a sudden, I realize I am being supported. At times I seek contact through being in the moment and I become more conscious that there's a bigger power. I don't know all of "it" and probably never will. I just need to accept.

A number of years ago I began to realize, as I started my 500-hour yoga teacher training journey, that I was no longer just doing yoga/*asanas*; I was living yoga. I've been living yoga since then, it's just part of who I am now.

SPIRITUALITY IN YOGA

I believe yoga brings into my life the ability to be able to better understand myself, to be in the moment, to realize what's going on within my mind and my body. Maybe this is what spirituality is.

Susan Tebb
PhD, LSW, RYT-500, C-IAYT, USA

CHAPTER 9

Inner Guidance

This chapter presents six stories of profound journeys of self-discovery and spiritual awakening. Each narrative weaves a tapestry of personal transformation, highlighting the universal human quest for meaning and connection to something greater than ourselves. The stories begin in diverse settings—from the sun-baked plains of Nebraska to the bustling cities of Canada and Scotland. Despite their varied backgrounds, the individuals share a common thread: an innate sense that there's more to life than meets the eye.

THE VOICE

At age 27 I was pregnant with my son. There was unmeasurable joy within me during the whole nine months of pregnancy. I felt a new life slowly growing in me, and this was a perfect reason and purpose for my being. I lived now, in the moment! Pregnancy was a very deep spiritual experience, which gave me a very strong sense of *I am*.

The delivery of my son was normal; afterwards, however, I was heavily hemorrhaging and the doctor had difficulties stopping it. At a critical point I was suddenly overcome by this sweet, peaceful feeling. That's when for the first time I heard the inner Voice saying "All is okay. I delivered my son, and my husband can take care of him. I am free to go..." I was falling into a dark, sweet, and welcoming abyss of beingness. This total bliss lasted sometime, and then I came back to full awareness of nurses running around me in panic. About 12 months later, Raymond Moody's *Life After Life* popped into my hands, and there I found an explanation of my blissful state. And so now I know that *I am*, *I was*, and I always *will be*. The fear of death left me, and the veil became very thin.

I started meditating when I was 36, and with time my meditations became quite deep. One day I thought I heard a voice whispering into my ear. Then, from time to time, that whisper would come back during deeper meditations.

I didn't understand what the Voice was saying as the words were unrecognizable. But the whisper became quite intense with time and I couldn't disregard it anymore. I became quite concerned—was I going crazy?

A friend suggested that next time I heard the whisper I should ask that voice "Who are you?" In a few days I had an opportunity to ask in my mind "Who are you?" The voice whispered one word, which I immediately wrote down. I didn't know what it meant or what language it was in. Again, a friend suggested I should wait, and with time the answer would reveal itself to me.

A few months later, I was in the library with my son. As I walked around, I came to a shelf where a book attracted my attention. On impulse I pulled it out and opened it in the middle... And there it was! My word in Blackfoot language—The Great Spirit of the Indigenous Sioux tribe...

I stood there struck by the synchronicity of this, a sworn atheist, suddenly filled with fear. Right in the middle of Mississauga library I felt someone was saying "See... I do exist!" I was filled with knowing that I had been contacted by something Larger than life.

With time the Voice became more present in my life in the form of dialogue. At first it would concern major events. I was standing in the kitchen, preparing a meal during the day, when I heard "Cancer?"

"Not now, I am single parent!" someone within me answered. I stood there wondering who was asking and who was answering??!!

Then, a few years later, I was again standing in the kitchen preparing breakfast: "Cancer?" came the question again.

"No, not now!" something within me answered.

Again, I was left wondering, who was talking? Who was asking and who was answering?

The cancer came without any further questions a few years later.

In 2011 the Voice came back again—"Go to India to study yoga therapy!"

I had just recovered from a major health disaster, established myself as a yoga teacher, and I liked what I was doing. So why rock the boat?! But the more I resisted, the more obtrusive the Voice became. Finally, I gave in and signed up for a nine-month course at the Kaivalyadhama Yoga Institute in India. Little did I know that I would stay there six years!

While at Kaivalyadhama I was asked to do research on yoga and cancer. As I thought about it, the Voice came: "You will design a protocol for a rehabilitation and recovery program after cancer treatment, based on your own experience with cancer. You will include *asana*, *pranayama*, meditation, *yoga nidra*, *mudras*, chanting, and cleansing practices."

In 15 minutes I "downloaded" the whole protocol. This is how the Beyond Cancer program was born. Consequently, the CEO asked me to stay at Kaivalyadhama as a senior yoga therapist and run Beyond Cancer retreats. I did this for six years, witnessing the miraculous healings of hundreds of cancer patients.

Interestingly, I had to gradually grow my trust in this inner guidance. It started with a very quiet voice asking me to do something small. As I listened and followed its guidance, the directions would increase in either perceived difficulty or even absurdity. It came to a perhaps most astonishing directive when I felt I had to jump into what seemed like an impossible situation. As I hesitated and disputed the action in front of me, the Voice said "Are you ready to walk the talk or just talk the talk?!" I had no choice but do what I was told to do—with great and unexpected results.

As time passed, the more I cleared my own "impurities" (*kleshas*) and conditioning by observing my daily *sadhana*, the clearer and louder was the "small still Voice" within me. With time my "conversations" with the Voice became a normal occurrence. *It* became my mentor and my trusted "go to" guide. To follow its lead sometimes seemed illogical, sometimes irrational, or even risky—as the directions occasionally felt outrageous. Yet, every time I followed this Voice, it led to positive results, not only for me, but for everyone who was concerned.

Since then, I have stopped questioning the instructions and simply follow them, trusting and knowing that the next steps will be revealed to me at the right time. I have been led to places, people, and situations I would never have been able to imagine in my wildest dreams. As the connection with my Voice grows, so does my inner peace and well-being, too. I now know that I do not have to worry about anything, I do not have to know anything ahead of time. The right solutions or words come in the moment when they are needed. And if I want to move in the wrong direction, I am immediately notified, with an alternative choice offered. All I have to do is simply "rest in my being," "listen," and through my *sadhana* keep working on deepening my connection to the Voice.

Yogacharini Lee Majewski
MA, C-IAYT, C-IYA, Author and Founding Director
of the Yoga for Health Institute, USA

FROM DIVERSE ROOTS TO INNER GUIDANCE

Growing up on the sun-baked plains of Western Nebraska, my relationship with God started in an unusual way. Our family was deeply rooted in Methodist Christianity. My mother's family were also Methodists; her mother was deeply suspicious of Catholics. My grandfather served as a Ku Klux Klan member. The Klan in that town left Black people alone and were mostly after the Catholics. Yet despite this rigid Protestant upbringing, something else called to me.

In my childhood bedroom, around age eight or nine, I kept a secret altar. While other kids my age were playing with toys, I found myself drawn to the mystical beauty of the Eucharist, a fascination that would have surely raised eyebrows in my Protestant household.

Television became my window to a broader spiritual world. I found myself captivated by Bishop Sheen, a Catholic evangelist whose charismatic presence on TV spoke to something deep within me. The Catholic mass, with its rich traditions and rituals, held me spellbound. During my teenage years, my world expanded further as we explored meditation, Hindu practices, and Buddhism in social studies. A seed was planted—a recognition that spiritual truth might lie beyond the boundaries of any single tradition.

My life took a significant turn in high school through debate club. Our coach, who taught Humanities, arranged for a Hindu priest to visit our class one Thursday. The moment he began speaking about meditation, something awakened in me. His lecture transcended mere academic discourse—it was as if a door to a new dimension had opened. When he explained how Catholic mass contained tantric elements, my spiritual puzzle pieces began falling into place.

At 16, first love brought another dimension to my spiritual journey. It wasn't just teenage romance; it was a gateway to something profound. Between the ages of 16 and 19, extraordinary things began happening. I developed an uncanny ability to visualize my boyfriend's face and sense his location with inexplicable accuracy. During one meditation, I entered a space of pure joy that felt otherworldly. Time seemed to stop, and in that crystalline moment, I heard a voiceless voice declare, "Your life will be for love." Although I couldn't fully grasp its significance then, this message would become my life's mission.

My quest led me through meditation classes and spiritual organizations. I explored ancient Asian wisdom traditions. I delved into Sanskrit under Swami Veda's guidance and Swami Rama became my guru. Yet something was still missing. Initially drawn to medicine, I began working as a nursing assistant and started pre-med courses. But life had other plans.

After three years in a row of good grades and several rounds of rejection from medical schools, a profound realization struck—this wasn't my path. The universe seemed to whisper that my calling lay elsewhere. When I discovered clinical psychology, particularly through a Catholic university program, everything aligned. Here was a way to blend my spiritual understanding with practical service to others.

In my 20s, I was still dealing with all of the confusion and depression around being gay. As a way out of depression I decided to challenge myself: I should learn to climb a really high mountain and conquer my fear of heights—that would be a big deal! I signed up for a mountaineering course and I fell totally in love with mountaineering. I didn't realize that I had set up a real crisis for myself.

One year, in Peru, while climbing in the Andes, all of a sudden these giant pinnacles of ice started to poke up out of the horizon, and it scared me to death. As we made base camp I was getting more and more anxious every minute. After a sleepless night we were off to an advance climb. At one point I turned a corner—here is this fantastic peak, just shy of 6000 meters. I can see it in my mind even now. It had a glacier on top that tumbled all the way down to the base. About every 10 minutes icebergs would calve off the glacier and fall into the lake. While I'm passing by, one of these happened next to me, and I'm just absolutely dumbstruck with the beauty of it. It interrupted my whole anxious thought process, just sort of kicked it off my head. And there was this atmosphere of heaven and suddenly I'm just completely surrounded by beauty. The voice comes—*I am always with you!*

What I learned in retrospect up there was to think of my fear of heights as an alarm system. It's something to alert you to when you're in danger. Also, it took me a long time to realize that, in retrospect, this was the voice of my guru. It didn't sound like him. My inner contact with my guru is very soft, motherly, very quiet. It really is the still, small voice of the *Old Testament*. I feel I am being led. I feel led at this point in my life into a larger sense of living a mindful life. It's not so much about the time I sit down and meditate anymore. I still do that. But it's really about, where is your mind?

I look back and I have this feeling of presence in me. The presence of my guru, Swami Rama, and of Swami Veda, that I realize now has been there from childhood, from those early days of sitting in church and wondering, what is this feeling up above my head? When did my spiritual quest start? I think that sense of presence is a really good answer. If meditation is about anything, it's about teaching your mind—listen, really listen. I think that sense of listening to presence is what I would identify as the first thing on the spiritual path.

Looking back now, I see how each step, each seemingly random encounter, was part of a greater design. From that secret altar in my childhood bedroom to my present work in psychology, my journey has been a continuous unfolding of that early message: a life dedicated to love, understanding, and the bridge between spiritual wisdom and human experience.

The Protestant child who kept a hidden altar grew into someone who learned to embrace the vast tapestry of spiritual truth, finding beauty in both Eastern and Western traditions. My story isn't about leaving one faith for another; it's about discovering how all paths can lead to the same divine understanding, when approached with an open heart and a curious mind.

Stephen (Stoma) Parker
PsyD, Emeritus Psychologist, C-IAYT, E-RYT-500, YACEP, USA

FROM IRISH CATHOLIC ROOTS TO SPIRITUAL TEACHER

I never imagined my path from Irish Catholic roots to spiritual teacher would take so many twists and turns. Growing up in Scotland after my father's early death, I was immersed in Catholic tradition—the rituals, confessions, and the everyday support and guidance of priests in the lives of people in our community. While I loved the stories and mythology as a child, my teenage years brought difficult questions about doctrine that went unanswered. The church and the community, once comforting, began to feel more set up to hold people in unquestioning obedience and acquiescence, and my modern, commonsense concerns about women's rights and empowerment were burning, and I needed to find a philosophy that was more suited to who I felt myself to be.

Life took a dark turn as my mother's alcoholism deepened and my own addiction emerged. Despite outward success in my corporate career, I was dying inside. The salary and job security I had studied for and worked hard to attain became a hollow refuge from the emotional chaos within. Multiple suicide attempts and ICU visits left me empty and desperate. I was fired from my job and decided to take a year off in California, to sort myself out.

Within nine months of moving to the USA, my life was again a wreck. I woke up one day, severely hungover and fired from another job, with the familiar idea of suicide. However, alongside that old voice was a calm yet insistent suggestion that I simply go to an AA meeting. It wasn't dramatic or mystical, just a quiet knowing that I had to choose life. The voice was gentle, but firm, like a mother calling her child home. In that moment of clarity, I realized that all my years of running had led me right back to myself.

Early sobriety brought its own challenges. The thought of re-entering corporate life twisted my stomach into knots. My soul was crying out for something more authentic, something deeper. I returned to a *Hatha Yoga* practice—I had taken classes at the Sivananda Yoga Centre in London. Those initial classes had always connected me with something deep and profound—especially in *shavasana*, where I could actually experience, as a felt sensation within me, an inner sanctuary and sense of purpose, a possibility of meaning and strength in this life.

The real transformation began when I heard Mark Halpern speak about Ayurveda at the Sivananda Yoga Farm in California. It was like every cell in my body resonated with truth. The ancient wisdom he shared spoke directly to my heart with perfect resonance. Finally, I understood my purpose, my *dharma*—to bridge the worlds of recovery and holistic healing. This wasn't just about getting sober; it was about finding wholeness on every level—physical, mental, emotional, and spiritual.

My journey became about integrating these ancient wisdom traditions with modern recovery. I immersed myself in study, traveling to India, sitting with teachers, and, most importantly, practicing what I learned. The more I practiced, the more I understood that addiction wasn't just about substances; it was about disconnection from our true nature. The work isn't always easy. Sometimes it means sitting with clients in their darkness, holding space as they find their own light. I've learned to be comfortable with silence, with tears, with the raw vulnerability of souls on healing journeys.

Each day brought new insights. I discovered that the Catholic rituals of my childhood weren't so different from the Sanskrit mantras I now chanted. Both were pathways to the Divine, different languages speaking the same truth. The Virgin Mary and goddess Durga began to merge in my understanding—different faces of the Divine Mother who had been guiding me all along.

Today, my practice centers on mantra and maintaining that vital connection to Spirit. I've learned that spirituality isn't about dramatic revelations; it's about showing up each day, taking a few conscious breaths, and trusting the process. It's about finding the sacred in the ordinary—in the steam rising from my morning tea, in the way sunlight filters through leaves, in the grateful tears of a client who's finally found their way home.

The greatest gift has been watching others discover their own path to healing, whether through physical *asana* practice or deeper spiritual inquiry. I see myself in their struggles, in their moments of doubt and breakthrough. Each success story reminds me of that hospital room where my own life could so easily have ended, and I'm filled with gratitude for the path that led me here.

What began as a desperate attempt to save myself has blossomed into a life's purpose. Every challenge, every dark night of the soul, has served to deepen my understanding and compassion. The programs I've developed combining the multiple recovery pathways (including 12 steps) with yoga therapy have reached people I never thought possible. Sometimes, when I'm teaching, I catch glimpses of my younger self in the participants' eyes—that same longing for wholeness, that same spark of hope.

Now I can truly say that recovery isn't just about staying sober; it's about coming home to ourselves, one breath, one moment, one awakening at a time. It's about remembering who we really are beneath the layers of conditioning and pain. Each morning, as I light a candle and sit for meditation, I feel the presence of all those who have helped me along the way—my Catholic ancestors, my yoga teachers, my AA sponsors, and most of all, my mother, whose struggle with alcoholism led to her untimely death and ultimately led me to this path of service.

As I continue this journey, I remain humbled by the wisdom that unfolds daily. The Irish Catholic girl who once questioned everything has found her answers not in dogma, but in the living experience of Spirit moving through every aspect of life. This is the message I share: trust the journey, even when you can't see the path ahead. The light within never dim; sometimes we just need help remembering how to access it.

And in those quiet moments between breaths, between thoughts, between the spaces of doing and being, I know with absolute certainty that I am exactly where I'm meant to be. The path continues to unfold, one day, one step at a time, leading me ever deeper into the mystery of healing and transformation.

Durga Leela
BA, AP-NAMA, C-IAYT, eRYT Founder and
Author of Yoga of Recovery, *USA*

FINDING MY WAY HOME

I've always known there was something more. Even as a child of nine or ten, I remember lying in bed, contemplating mortality with a certainty that defied my young age. "I'm not going to die," I would think, not out of childish denial, but from a deep, inexplicable knowing. I couldn't articulate it then, but I was connecting with something eternal within me—that essence that has always been here and will never not be here.

Looking back now, I can trace the breadcrumbs of my spiritual journey through seemingly ordinary moments. In college, when I was terrified of flying to Sweden for my study abroad program, an older woman taught me visualization. "See yourself on the plane," she said. "Imagine yourself arriving with your group." I didn't know then that I was practicing *bhavana*, but that simple technique opened my eyes to new ways of being in the world.

Even my peculiar bedtime ritual as a teenager—talking to my body parts, telling them one by one to "go to sleep"—was actually a form of body scanning. These practices came naturally to me, bubbling up from some inner wisdom I didn't yet understand. It wasn't until years later, studying yoga therapy and *yoga nidra*, that I recognized these early intuitive connections for what they were.

My formal yoga journey began in my early 30s, taking classes in an old lighthouse for back pain, and then later while pregnant in a home studio. As my children grew older, I thought, "Why not take a teacher training? Just for me." But that first taste only awakened my hunger for deeper understanding. I found myself enrolled in a yoga therapy program at LMU (Loyola Marymount University), driven by an insatiable need to understand more than just the superficial anatomy and physiology. I've always needed to be really good at something before teaching it—it's just who I am.

The transformative power of *pranayama* captured me completely. Each practice brought a deeper settling, a profound connection to myself, and a quiet peace that left me wanting more. This led me to explore iRest *yoga nidra*, a self-inquiry practice where I experienced moments of pure transcendence. I found myself entering a spacious openness that wasn't sleep but something far more refreshing and profound.

Today, I've developed the capacity to rest in witnessing presence, observing my behaviors, thoughts, and emotions. Don't get me wrong—I'm still beautifully human. I say things I wish I hadn't, and catch myself in negative self-talk, but now I can notice these patterns with kindness. "Oh, you're doing that again!" I'll think, with a gentle smile rather than judgment.

Teaching has become my own form of learning. I light up when sharing these practices, feeling excitement bubble up from my core. My personal *sadhana* has evolved beyond formal practice times, spilling into everyday moments of mindful awareness. The *yamas* and *niyamas* are constant companions, coloring how I move through the world.

Yet I still struggle sometimes. My cognitive mind often overrides my heart's wisdom, and I battle with imposter syndrome. Who am I, a middle-aged white woman, to teach these ancient Eastern practices? I wrestle with questions of cultural appropriation and authenticity, always striving to be respectful and careful with these precious teachings.

In my work with clients, relationship is everything. I want them to feel seen and heard, creating a safe space for reconnection with themselves. So many issues stem from broken relationships—with others and with ourselves. I practice careful listening and gentle reframing, helping people move from judgment to neutral observation. Instead of a "bad knee" we might say "a knee that hurts right now."

The spiritual element of yoga remains, for me, its most profound gift. It saddens me that many don't realize this deeper dimension exists. In my deepest knowing, I understand that we are all whole and complete—heart meeting heart, essence meeting essence. While I intellectually grasp this truth, I'm still on the journey of fully embodying it. And perhaps that's exactly as it should be.

Every day brings new opportunities for curiosity and growth. I find myself constantly asking, "What is happening here? What is this sensation? What can I learn from this moment?" My practice has become less about achieving perfect poses and more about cultivating presence and awareness in every breath.

When I look back at that little girl who couldn't imagine not existing, I smile at her intuitive wisdom. She knew something that would take me decades to fully understand—that beneath all our doing and thinking and struggling, there exists an unchanging essence, a spark of the divine that never dims. This is the truth I live and teach, one breath, one student, one moment at a time.

Laurie Angress
C-IAYT, Certified Yoga Therapist, iRest Meditation Instructor, USA

A PHYSIOTHERAPIST'S JOURNEY: FROM CONVENTIONAL PRACTICE TO EMBRACING ENERGY HEALING AND SUBTLE BODY AWARENESS

After about 15 years as a physiotherapist with a specialization in manual therapy and chronic pain, I had an experience that transformed my understanding of the body and profoundly changed the way I work as a physiotherapist and yoga therapist.

During my early years as a physiotherapist, the predominant theory was that movement impairments and pain were due to injury or disease of the structure of the body. My expertise was in identifying the physical dysfunction and then "fixing" it. While this undoubtably helped thousands of patients, it often was not sufficient in helping those with persistent pain.

One such patient with a long history of chronic pain had a session with an energy healer named Kate. The session was focused on the client's emotional blockages, yet the "physical" effects of that energy healing session were undeniable. I was intrigued by the profound improvement in "physical" pain this patient received during the energy healing session, so I booked a session for myself to see what it was all about.

Kate had me lie supine on a massage table and practice "shamanic breathing." Very quickly, I felt a flood of emotions and Kate began to guide me in tuning into these emotional sensations. After about 15 minutes I repositioned my left leg and explained that the supine position caused numbness in my thigh due to a 15-year old psoas injury with femoral nerve adhesions.

A diagnostic ultrasound and MRI confirmed that the psoas had tears and there was scarring that had impeded the mobility of the femoral nerve. I saw no connection between the emotions that we were exploring and what I understood to be positional discomfort in my leg. Kate, however, was convinced that any symptom that arose during the session was energetically connected. We continued the session with visualization, breath, and compassionate listening to this region in my hip. At the end of the session, the black blob I had visualized in the region of the psoas had traveled down my left leg and out my foot, and along with it went both the difficult emotions and the physical "nerve" symptoms. Since that day I have been able to lie supine without pain.

Over the years, understanding of the mind–body connection has evolved in the field; however, the concept of an "energetic body" remains elusive. Modern science, as of yet, is unable to quantify or qualify such a concept. To appease my academic mind, I had a repeat diagnostic ultrasound, which remained unchanged from prior imaging. Kate explained that the issue was stagnant energy from an unresolved emotional trauma. By moving the energy through mindful intention and breath, the blockage had cleared and the pain disappeared.

In 2005 I joined Kate on a journey to visit the pre-historic Goddess Temples of Malta. During a visit to the Ħal Saflieni Hypogeum, skepticism was replaced with deep conviction, and my perspective on the human experience was profoundly transformed. While visiting this ancient neolithic site, which dates back to 4000 to 2500 BCE, I felt a sense of centrifugal force pulling me into the earth. Then, I sensed the presence of a woman massively larger than any human. My left hand was on a large rock and my head lifted towards this mystical presence. I was feeling intense vibration coursing from the rock through my left hand, up my arm, and through my body. I sensed that I was receiving a download that was not comprehensible by the mind. It was as if electrical energy was transmitting from the rocks into my body, and my body knew what to do. I had not yet processed all that occurred, and yet I knew something in me had changed.

After this experience my yoga practice shifted from focusing on mechanical alignment and breath to the more subtle awareness of *pranic* flow. Most of the patients I treated wanted me to "fix them" with manual therapy or teach them yoga *asana* to "fix" their injuries. This "gross" body emphasis seemed less important, especially for those with persistent pain. Instead, I sensed energetic blockages, psychophysiological connections, and alterations in body awareness. After a few "miracle" cases such as a client suddenly being able to walk again, I conducted a pilot study to try to understand the subtle body. While all those in the experimental group had significant improvement, I realized that it may simply not be explainable yet from a modern science perspective.

Thirteen years later, at the bedside of my father as he was actively dying, I reached for his hand and felt the same sense of electricity coursing from his hand through mine and up my arm. The sensation was viscerally familiar to the electrical vibration I felt deep underground in Malta. Then his eyes closed, and as the vibration intensified, I felt the same sense of expansive peace and trust I had experienced in the Hypogeum. After the vibration stopped, his body's death process accelerated. I know now, beyond doubt, that the subtle body is real and that there is so much more that modern science has yet to comprehend.

This experience seemed to shift something in me, something I cannot explain. The experience of *prana* transcended the thinking mind. On a practical level I lost interest in trying to figure it out. The experience also gifted me with a profound sense of interconnectedness and love.

I understand now that as a yoga therapist it is not my place to push my perspective onto my clients. My job now is to understand their perspective and offer them practices without attachment to the outcome. I no longer feel that I am fixing or healing anyone. I believe that the essence of yoga therapy is to attune to that which opens the client to their wholeness and shifts away from identification with dis-ease. Attuning myself and my clients to spiritual connection with something bigger, something beyond what we can perceive, is where the healing comes from.

It is in this space of spiritual connection where I find peace and contentment, especially during the most difficult of times. I hold a strong conviction that everyone has the capacity to cultivate such inner peace. Transformative life experiences, such as what I experienced in Malta and with my father, "woke me up." And my daily *sadhana* nurtures that which awoke. This enables me to support my clients in their own unique awakening.

Lori Rubenstein Fazzio
DPT, PT, MAppSc, C-IAYT, C-IYA, Clinical Professor of Yoga and Health, Loyola Marymount University Graduate Yoga Studies, Bellarmine College of Liberal Arts, USA

A PATH OF DIVERSE INFLUENCES AND INNER GUIDANCE

I come from a diverse and eclectic family. My grandparents on my mother's side are/were Japanese Buddhists while my father's parents were Anglican. As a child my parents were best described as agnostics who hedged their bets by sending my brother and I to a Japanese nondenominational evangelical Sunday School without them. This diversity sparked my curiosity about belief and faith from an early age.

A pivotal moment in my spiritual journey came when I was 12. Watching television with my grandmother, which was our afterschool ritual, I saw Deepak Chopra discuss *chakras*. It resonated deeply with me, especially given my struggles with chronic strep throat and feeling unheard. This inner recognition of truth and falsehood became a guiding principle in my life.

My undergraduate degree in Religion and Modern Thought at the University of Toronto further fueled my fascination with belief systems. I wanted to understand not just what people believe, but why they believe it and what needs it fulfills. This academic pursuit allowed me to explore spirituality through both intuitive and logical lenses.

My approach to spirituality has always been feeling the sense first, and then seeking validation. Leaps of faith guided my youth. For example, when my aunt showed me an ad for teacher's education in Australia, I felt the universe guiding me there. It was a leap of faith, but I followed that inner guidance. I discovered Ayurveda at 23, just after leaving Canada, and became fascinated by it.

In Australia, my first job as a teacher beautifully merged English and Religious Studies, allowing for spiritual conversations within the confines of curriculum. I reached out to Buddhist monks and other spiritual figures, inviting them to share their life journeys with students. This experience, along with my practicum supervisor being an officiant, felt like synchronicity, aligning with my desire to be part of life's significant moments.

Throughout my journey I've learned to pause and reflect deeply when at a crossroads, trusting that if I'm on the right path, the universe will let it unfold. I've made mistakes, sometimes losing my way when I stop listening, trusting, or surrendering. In these moments, I engage in long internal dialogues, often during walks. I'm not sure who's answering my questions, but I'm comfortable with that uncertainty.

When life becomes chaotic and my ability to receive or interpret messages wanes, I create *tapas*—a space of complete stillness and nothingness. This reset allows me to reconstruct aspects of myself or my identity. My move to Australia was part of this process, providing a new environment conducive to growth and self-discovery.

I've come to realize that sometimes I need to return to complete stillness to regrow myself. This practice of stepping back, resetting, and then moving forward has been a powerful tool in my spiritual journey, allowing me to maintain my connection to inner guidance and continue growing on my path. This commitment to a path of lifelong learning is something I am to share in my work as an educator, yoga therapist, and metaphysical minister.

Reverend Danielle Atkinson
OCT, C-IAYT, E-RYT-500, CAHP/CCA, Ayurvedic Professional Canada,
Clinical Professor of Yoga and Health, Loyola Marymount University,
Graduate Yoga Studies, Bellarmine College of Liberal Arts, USA

CHAPTER 10

Seeking Out

The path to spiritual awakening rarely follows a straight line. Through these seven intimate narratives, we see how different individuals—from scientists to military officers to academics—found their way to deeper spiritual understanding through widely varying routes. Some began as sensitive children naturally attuned to mystical experiences while others stumbled into spirituality through unexpected channels such as psychedelics or personal crisis. What emerges is a tapestry of transformation, where early experiences often planted seeds that would flower years later.

FROM SENSITIVITY TO SPIRITUALITY: A JOURNEY OF CONNECTION AND SERVICE

As I reflect on my life, I'm reminded of the sensitivity that has been a part of me since childhood. Growing up, I was often told to "dial it down," as if my heightened awareness of the world around me was somehow too much. But this sensitivity, I now realize, was the foundation of my spiritual path.

My early years were spent in close communion with nature. I didn't see myself as separate from the natural world; instead, I felt deeply connected to everything around me. This connection was nurtured by my parents, who embodied a unique blend of community service and an appreciation for beauty.

However, it was a profound and terrifying experience at the age of 11 that truly set my spiritual journey in motion. Attending a friend's church gathering, I found myself in the midst of what I can only describe as a spiritual occupation. Lying on the ground, I began speaking "in tongues;" words and sounds pouring from me that I had no command over. The crowd watched in awe, but for me, it was a moment of sheer panic. There was no context, no guidance, and no one to help me understand what was happening.

This experience, as powerful as it was, initially pushed me away from spirituality. The church leaders saw me as a potential "channel," but I was overwhelmed and frightened. In a moment of rebellion against this intense and uncontrolled experience, I rejected religion and spirituality altogether. I remember having a conversation with God, saying, "If this is what connecting with you means, I don't want it."

Deep down, however, I knew there was more to existence than just this physical realm. I couldn't shake the feeling that we weren't meant to be isolated beings moving through a single lifetime. This underlying longing eventually led me to yoga in my early 20s.

Yoga changed everything for me. It allowed me to engage with spirituality in a way that felt safe. I learned to modulate my experiences, and to reach beyond myself without losing myself or feeling overwhelmed. It provided a framework for my embodied research, and allowed me to access spiritual realms while remaining grounded in my body.

As I delved deeper into yoga, I found myself drawn to yoga therapy. This path aligned more closely with my innate sensitivity and desire to help others. It stood in stark contrast to my earlier work in sports psychology, where I often felt conflicted about participating with athletes who had to push themselves beyond their physical limits for the sake of performance.

In my practice as a yoga therapist, I've come to recognize and trust a generous supportive wisdom that seems readily available. When working with clients, I often hear an inner voice guiding me, suggesting approaches or insights that I wouldn't have consciously considered. At first, I was hesitant to trust these promptings, but I've learned that when I bring them to my clients to consider, they invariably prove helpful. Even when guiding a yoga class, I notice that the words coming out of my mouth are not entirely my own. There's a steady and kind partnership, or co-creation, if only I can soften to it.

This sense of deep connection or union has always been there, even if I didn't recognize it or understand it. The experience of having children deepened my spiritual inquiry and trust, reinforcing my belief that there's more to life than the obvious biology. I came to see my role as a parent as part of a larger spiritual relationship, with these beings temporarily entrusted to my care for reasons beyond my full comprehension.

As I've grown in my spiritual practice, I've come to see this connection as a relationship that requires tending. It's not just about receiving guidance or wisdom; it's about reciprocity—offering praise, gratitude, and service in return. Although this animate and loving force isn't something I can name or fully define, I've learned to trust it implicitly.

Working with people who are dying has been a profound aspect of my spiritual learning. Far from being stressful or depressing, I find it to be a great privilege and honor. It brings me closer to the great mystery of existence, and allows me to engage with the deepest aspects of human experience. This work has shown me that spirituality isn't only about stress relief or personal wellness; it seems to be more about learning to be a faithful witness and yielding to life herself.

My recent focus on aging has further expanded my understanding of spirituality's role in life. Through lived experience, clinical research, and teaching at the university, I've observed how society influences people's perspectives on aging and purpose in later life. It's been eye-opening to see how some cultures view retirement as a time of personal indulgence, while others see it as an opportunity for continued service and contribution to future generations.

This cultural divide highlights a wise consideration of *dharma*, not only as a personal purpose but as a way of tending to community. I've come to see that individualism pales to the call of serving the greater good, both in living and in how one comes to their dying days.

Reflecting on my life, I realize how much yoga has informed and guided me. It has provided a rich framework for an enduring wonderment and a way to explore spirituality that is gratefully received. Yoga philosophy presents a sense of accompaniment, connecting me to a long lineage of seekers who have wrestled with similar existential questions.

Yoga has given me a community, a map, and an ever-changing practice. I rarely have the feeling of being lonely or lost. As I practice going within, I'm in conversation with all the uncertainties and deep mysteries of life, and it is not at all unsettling. The daily walk on the path only asks me to be present and attentive, and to offer myself to others and what is needed in each alive moment, trusting I'm not traveling alone.

Anne Pitman
MSc, C-IAYT, Director of the School of Embodied Yoga Therapy,
Associate Professor at the University of Ottawa, Canada

A JOURNEY THROUGH SERVICE AND SPIRIT

I can't really remember a time when spirituality wasn't woven into the fabric of my existence. In my family, spirituality was as natural as breathing, an inheritance that shaped my understanding of the vast universe that we are part of.

There has always been a constant awareness that there is more than what meets the eye, more than our limited human comprehension can grasp.

Growing up in West Texas, I was fortunate that my parents created a protective bubble around me and my brothers that somehow shielded us from many of the harshest realities of racial segregation and discrimination. This early foundation of security allowed my spiritual nature to flourish naturally, untainted by the prejudices that existed beyond our community.

At around the age of eight or nine, I went through the questioning phase that many children experience. How could I believe in something I couldn't see, touch, or feel? These questions lingered as I went to college, where exposure to different cultures and perspectives broadened my understanding of spirituality. The beauty was in discovering how others approached their spiritual journeys with such openness.

My military career spanning 26 years brought its own set of spiritual lessons. In the face of gender and racial challenges, I maintained my perspective: treating everyone with kindness until they showed me that I needed to adjust my approach. There were countless moments of divine intervention that I can't explain, situations where I felt protected by something greater than myself. Even in the most dangerous situations, my thought was simple—if today was my day to go, I needed to ensure I'd done what I needed to do.

One particularly memorable experience occurred in Bergen, Norway. I spent hours atop a mountain overlooking fjords, absorbing a view that would become my meditation anchor for years to come. The clouds hovering above the mountains, the panoramic vista below—it was a moment of pure connection with something greater than myself. To this day, when I close my eyes to meditate, I return to that peaceful scene.

Throughout my military service, I faced challenges related to both gender and race. Yet, I approached each situation with the same philosophy—I would treat everyone with kindness until they proved that wasn't the path forward. This approach wasn't always easy, especially when confronted with direct discrimination, like the time I was told that women weren't smart enough to be officers. Instead of anger, I chose to follow my path. It was a path that proved the naysayers wrong.

For me, God is the name I give to this greater power, and I acknowledge there's an expanse of consciousness in the universe that my brain can't fully grasp. I don't always know when God is working through me, but I trust that my intentions—seeking to do no harm and looking to be helpful—align with divine purpose. Sometimes I've even said things that surprised myself, making me wonder, "Where did that come from?"

My journey into yoga came through a friend's invitation, and while I found physical challenges, I also discovered a philosophy that resonated with my existing spiritual framework. There were moments when I needed to reconcile yoga's philosophical aspects with my own beliefs, particularly regarding the concept of multiple deities versus my nondual belief in one God. But I've learned to acknowledge that there are many paths through life, even if they differ from my own.

In my work as a yoga therapist, I've learned to meet clients where they are on their spiritual journey. Some find their connection to the divine on the golf course, others in nature, and some prefer not to acknowledge spirituality at all. That's okay—they still move in it, even if they don't recognize it. During intake conversations, I gauge their comfort level with spirituality and adjust my approach accordingly.

I've experienced profound moments of connection, particularly during *yoga nidra*, where time, space, and substance dissolve into pure consciousness. These experiences of equanimity, like a blank canvas where you touch your own consciousness, remind me of the vastness of spiritual existence. Yet, I don't chase after these experiences; I trust that they will come when needed.

My mother, who holds a ThD in Theology, has been a wonderful spiritual conversation partner. Our discussions have helped me evolve from questioning the reality of the divine to fully embracing the faith that there is something far greater than what we can comprehend. The questions have changed from "Is it real?" to a deep appreciation for the infinite nature of the divine that exists beyond our human understanding.

Through all my experiences—military service, yoga practice, and personal spiritual journey—I've come to understand that spirituality isn't about having all the answers; it's about moving through life with awareness, being of service, and recognizing that we're all part of something greater than ourselves. Whether I'm teaching yoga, working with clients, or simply going about my daily life, I carry this understanding with me.

I consider myself a work in progress, always learning and growing. In my interactions with others, I recognize that spirituality manifests differently for everyone. My role isn't to impose my beliefs but to create a space where others can explore their own connection to the divine, whatever form that may take for them. This approach has allowed me to bridge gaps between different belief systems and to support others as they explore their own paths to spiritual understanding.

The journey continues to unfold, revealing new depths of understanding with each passing day. Through it all, I remain grateful for the spiritual foundation my parents provided, the experiences that have shaped my faith, and the opportunity to share this journey with others. In the end, it's not about reaching a destination but about remaining open to the divine presence that exists in every moment, in every person, and in every experience.

Marilyn Peppers-Citizen
PhD, MBA, NBC-HWC, E-RYT-500, C-IAYT, USA

A SCIENTIST'S JOURNEY FROM HALLUCINOGENS TO YOGA

My spiritual journey began in an unexpected way, during the countercultural movement of the late 1960s and early 1970s. As a curious 20-year-old with a scientific bent, I found myself drawn into the exploration of altered states of consciousness through hallucinogenic substances. Little did I know that this experimentation would set me on a lifelong path of spiritual discovery and growth.

My first profound mystical experience came through the use of these hallucinogenic substances. It was a state of deep, all-encompassing oneness—a dissolution of duality, where I felt I was everything and everything was me. The sense of peace, comfort, and blissful tranquility was unlike anything I had ever known. This experience fit the classic description of a mystical state, and it left an indelible mark on my psyche.

Driven by my scientific curiosity, I delved into the literature about these altered states of consciousness. A pivotal moment came when I discovered *The Master Game*, a book by Robert Sylvester de Ropp, a biochemist who had researched hallucinogens. He posited that while these substances could induce mystical states, relying on them could potentially rob the nervous system of its natural ability to produce such states. More importantly, he introduced me to the idea that these states could be achieved through natural means—specifically, through long-established contemplative practices like yoga and meditation.

This revelation opened up a whole new world for me. I began voraciously reading, discovering the entire field of human endeavor dedicated to pure spirituality, distinct from religiosity. I realized that achieving and practicing these states of consciousness could be a profound and meaningful life goal.

With this newfound purpose, I began my search for a meditation practice. As I explored various options, yoga stood out to me. Its holistic approach, incorporating physical postures, breathing techniques, relaxation, meditation, diet, and lifestyle, all focused towards spiritual growth, resonated deeply with my scientific mindset. It seemed logical that working on multiple behavioral practices would increase the likelihood of success in achieving these unitive states of consciousness.

Fate seemed to intervene when I discovered a yoga course at the University of Toronto. On the first day of class, I found myself face to face with a man in a white turban teaching *Kundalini Yoga*. This encounter led me to the local ashram, where I began attending classes and workshops, becoming increasingly involved with the practitioners and residents.

In July 1973, I took the plunge and moved into the ashram in Toronto. This marked the beginning of my immersion into a yoga lifestyle practice. While I never experienced the same intensity of mystical states that I had with hallucinogens, my yoga practice consistently brought me closer to that realm. I found myself experiencing a sense of peace, tranquility, joy, purpose, and meaning that grew stronger with regular practice.

Living in the ashram was a transformative experience on multiple levels. Beyond the individual practice, it introduced me to the challenges and growth opportunities of being part of a spiritual community. Interacting with a diverse group of individuals in close quarters taught me valuable lessons about relationships, conflict resolution, and personal growth.

The daily discipline of waking up at 4am for practice was challenging but immensely rewarding. These early morning sessions, filled with chanting and yoga alongside 30 other practitioners, created a powerful collective energy that fueled my spiritual growth. The practices built my resilience, increased my capacity to tolerate life's challenges, and provided a stable foundation of inner peace that I could always return to.

Throughout this journey, I was fortunate to have the guidance of Yogi Bhajan, my spiritual teacher, and I became a Sikh, as many of his students did. His insight and perception often surpassed my own, allowing him to see things in me and my life that I was blind to. His role as a spiritual teacher was to provide occasional guidance, helping me overcome my own limited vision, and steer me in the right direction when I veered off course. My personal experience of Yogi Bhajan's approach to spiritual guidance struck a balance between respecting his wisdom and maintaining individual responsibility. For me, his teaching emphasized looking to the inner guru, the consciousness within, rather than becoming overly dependent on an external authority, a construct that is central to Sikh spiritual philosophy.

As I progressed on this path, I came to understand that the gift of yoga extends far beyond physical benefits. It provides a behavioral strategy for navigating life's challenges with greater ease and resilience. The stability and tranquility I cultivated through my practice became a steady platform for making day-to-day life decisions. I learned that I could always return to that fundamental experience of who I really am, that deep unitive state, to find calm and clarity.

The intensity and frequency of practice can vary from person to person, but I've found that daily practice, ideally as part of a holistic yoga lifestyle, yields the most profound results. This lifestyle encompasses not just the formal practices, but also extends to diet, social interactions, career choices, ethics, and morality.

As I reflect on my decades-long journey, I realize that my initial experiences with hallucinogens and subsequent discovery of yoga set me on a path of lifelong learning and growth. While the specific practices and community structures have evolved over time, the core essence of the spiritual journey remains constant—the pursuit of that unitive state of consciousness, that deep sense of connection and peace.

Today, as I continue my own practice and contribute to scientific research on the benefits of yoga practices in specific populations and for specific conditions, I feel a responsibility to share these insights with others. I believe it's crucial to dispel misconceptions about yoga and meditation, helping people understand that these practices are neither exclusively religious nor purely physical. They are powerful tools for evolving one's state of consciousness and promoting holistic well-being, accessible to people of all ages, backgrounds, and physical capabilities.

My spiritual practice has unfolded as a gradual, ongoing process rather than a single dramatic event. It's a journey of continuous discovery, challenges, and growth. Through practice and open-minded exploration, I've come to experience a deeper sense of peace, purpose, and connection to the world around me. This path has not only transformed my personal life, but has also shaped my professional pursuits, allowing me to bridge the worlds of spiritual practice and scientific research.

Sat Bir Singh Khalsa
PhD, Associate Professor of Medicine, Harvard Medical School, USA

THE PATH WAS ALWAYS THERE

I was born seeing the world differently. Even at four years old, I would slip into spontaneous trance states, watching patterns on the ceiling of a car, or light moving horizontally between plants as I played for hours in the garden and sandbox. Nature spoke to me in ways I couldn't explain—I was a young mystic, conversing with plants, sensing energies others seemed blind to. My grandfather's deep spiritual presence during his nightly rosary prayers showed me what true devotion felt like. I could feel his aura, tangible and pure, especially during his Rosary prayers from 9 to 9:30pm every evening in the living room.

The pivotal moment came at 13 when I had a vision that would shape my entire life's direction. A wise man with a white beard, sun-darkened skin, and gentle wrinkles appeared to me, smiling down with knowing eyes for 30 minutes in the middle of the night. That image stayed with me for months, eventually leading me to explore ESP (extrasensory perception) and deeper spiritual studies. Even then, I understood something profound—that the world's problems stemmed from our individual inner states of evolution.

These spiritual experiences made me feel great within myself. I have always felt confident that God is present and active in our world. However, the times I asked others if they had ever experienced spiritual events, a confused silence accompanied by odd facial expressions was the response. I didn't know any spiritual types of people—everyone praised me for being Class President and a student athlete, but no one saw me for me. This caused me deep feelings of loneliness—as a kid surrounded by caring people, but still left me feeling unseen.

My journey in college commenced with "world peace" via international relations to a complete transformation in understanding human consciousness. During my time as an overseas student in Taiwan at 20, I met a swami who introduced me to classical yoga and meditation, practices I've maintained daily ever since. But it was in Japan where everything shifted. In a retreat center, I discovered that war wasn't just about politics; it was about our collective lack of enlightenment. This realization turned my focus from international relations to "internal relations."

The universe kept guiding me. One Japanese meditation mentor recognized something in me, noting how quickly I achieved advanced states. He directed me to India, to the Yoga Institute in Mumbai, where I met Dr. Jayadeva Yogendra. Those daily hour-long private sessions over the next six months while training to become a yoga therapist were preparing me for something I couldn't yet comprehend.

Then it happened—the *samadhi* experience. Four months into my stay,

Dr. Jayadeva facilitated my transition. I was pulled into a tunnel filled with the overwhelming sound of "Om," and then...nothing. Hours passed in what felt like timelessness. When I emerged, I had that stunned feeling, not fully comprehending what had happened. Memory is altered in these trance experiences. Days later a yoga student friend mentioned I had been glowing for the past few days. It was at that moment that my self-awareness was overwhelmed by the experience. It took four days to fully process what had occurred, but when I did, everything changed. The *Yoga Sutras*, once intellectual concepts, became living truths I could explain with the clarity of someone describing a game they'd just witnessed.

This direct experience transformed my understanding of yoga therapy. I realized that most practitioners were missing the essential spiritual core of yoga. The focus on *asana* and *pranayama* as primary healing tools seemed backwards to me. True healing comes from helping people connect with their deeper selves—the physical practices are beneficial, but secondary.

My path led me back to my own cultural roots through Dr. Jayadeva's gentle guidance. He suggested exploring Quakerism, recognizing that spiritual growth often flourishes in familiar soil. At the Quaker graduate school, I found my *dharma*—teaching yoga and providing spiritual direction to students. The 60 college students who came to my yoga classes weren't just learning *asanas*; they were discovering the *yamas* and *niyamas*, the ethical foundations of yoga.

Today, after decades of practicing yoga therapy, I see clearly that the magic of healing happens when we help people touch their spiritual essence. Physical relief may come through *asana*, but true freedom from suffering emerges when we realize our true nature. Every person I work with reminds me of that 13-year-old who saw the wise man, that 24-year-old in *samadhi*, that seeker who found his path.

I never took a conventional job because my *dharma* isn't a conventional calling. It's a recognition that we're all born with different levels of spiritual attunement, and my role is to help others discover and develop their own inner knowing. When I see someone grasp this truth—when their eyes light up with recognition of their own divine nature—I'm reminded of my grandfather's rosary prayers, of that glowing presence that first showed me what spiritual connection feels like.

I want to be clear that this journey has had many difficult times. Spiritual experiences are blissful, yet much hard work needs to happen on a daily basis. Spiritual practice requires facing personal weaknesses, accepting one's faults and still forging ahead. Completing a PhD in Yoga Therapy was hard, as the intellectual expansion seemed contrary to spiritual practice. Continuing to find my identity has been a lifelong journey. And when you have these deepfelt experiences of divinity, the witnessing of the world's suffering is not easy to manage.

These experiences that seemed to set me apart as a child now serve as bridges to help others find their way home to themselves. Every trance state, every vision, every moment of connection with nature prepared me for this work. It's not about teaching people something new; it's about helping them remember what their souls have always known.

Robert Butera
PhD, MDiv, PE, C-IAYT, Director of YogaLife Institute,
Comprehensive Yoga Therapy, USA

FROM SOUTHERN ROOTS TO HIMALAYAN HEIGHTS

Growing up in the Southern USA, I was born into a devout Protestant family where faith was an integral part of daily life. My earliest memories are infused with a sense of the divine, a connection that felt as natural as breathing. I recall pausing before opening Christmas presents to thank Jesus and wish him a happy birthday, a gesture that came from a place of genuine devotion rather than obligation.

My grandfather played a pivotal role in nurturing my spiritual curiosity. During our walks together, he would patiently explain the intricacies of our faith, answering my endless questions with wisdom and kindness. When I was just seven years old, my mother passed away, leaving a void that I instinctively sought to fill with an even deeper connection to God. Two years later, when my father remarried and went on his honeymoon, I asked my grandfather to help me formally join the church. Those daily walks became impromptu catechism lessons, cementing my bond with both my faith and my grandfather.

As I grew older, my spiritual journey took unexpected turns. My new stepmother belonged to the Church of Christ, a denomination that felt restrictive and alien to me. Our conflicting views on faith became a source of tension, particularly during my teenage years. I found myself yearning for the familiar comfort of my childhood church, often pleading to attend services there instead of accompanying my family to their new place of worship.

My college years at Emory University in Atlanta marked a significant shift in my spiritual perspective. Studying religion and philosophy opened my eyes to a vast world of beliefs and ideologies. I was particularly drawn to Gnosticism and began to question the rigid structures of my childhood faith. The diverse student body, including many Jewish classmates, further expanded my understanding of different spiritual traditions.

After completing my PhD I moved to Chicago with my husband, where I was introduced to yoga by a close friend. This first encounter with Eastern spirituality was both intriguing and overwhelming. The physical practice resonated with me, but the vegetarian diet, chanting, and unfamiliar philosophy felt foreign. However, the seed had been planted.

When we relocated to Colorado, I found myself in a hotbed of spiritual alternatives. The rugged beauty of the Rockies awakened a deep appreciation for nature-based spirituality, and I began exploring Native American traditions. Simultaneously, I delved into Buddhism and rekindled my interest in yoga. It was during this period of exploration that I attended a yoga conference in Estes Park and met Rod Stryker, a teacher who would profoundly influence my spiritual path.

Stryker's approach to yoga was comprehensive, integrating *asana* practice with *pranayama*, meditation, and philosophy. This holistic method resonated deeply with me, offering a bridge between the physical and the spiritual that I had been seeking. I began studying with him regularly, attending retreats and workshops that would shape the next two decades of my life.

One pivotal moment came during a retreat in Maui when I was 40 years old. It was shortly after the 9/11 attacks, and the world felt uncertain and frightening. This retreat became a sanctuary, a place to reconnect with my Inner Self and the Divine. The experience was so transformative that I decided to pursue teacher training with Stryker, deepening my commitment to yoga as both a practice and a spiritual path. As I immersed myself in yoga philosophy, I found a new way of understanding the Divine that felt more aligned with my evolving beliefs. The concept of God shifted from an anthropomorphic figure to a universal wisdom, present in all things. I was particularly drawn to the balance of masculine and feminine energies in yogic thought, a stark contrast to the patriarchal structure of my childhood faith.

My spiritual home became the Himalayan Institute in Pennsylvania, where I would regularly attend retreats and trainings. These experiences, combined with my ongoing studies with Stryker, provided a steady, grounding presence in my life.

One particularly poignant moment in my spiritual journey came when I was preparing for my first trip to India with the Himalayan Institute. Just days before my departure, my husband unexpectedly lost his job, our beloved cat passed away, and the world was reeling from a terrorist threat that changed air travel forever. Amidst this chaos, I found myself on a plane to India, feeling lost and alone.

However, it was in this moment of despair that I experienced a profound sense of connection and support. Fellow travelers from the Himalayan Institute, strangers until that moment, offered comfort and assistance. This act of kindness reminded me of the interconnectedness of all beings, a central tenet of the spiritual path I had chosen.

The pilgrimage through the Himalayas that followed was a transformative experience. Visiting ancient temples and sacred sites, I felt a deep resonance with the spiritual energy of the land. The challenges of the journey—the altitude, the physical exertion, the unfamiliar surroundings—all served to bring me closer to the divine presence I had always sensed.

Reflecting on my spiritual journey, I realize it has been characterized not by dramatic, mystical experiences, but by a growing, steady sense of Divine presence and connection. It's a deep-felt belief that has become more refined and nuanced over time, informing every aspect of my life.

My journey has taught me that spirituality is not about adhering to a set of rigid beliefs or practices, but about cultivating a relationship with the Divine that is authentic and personal. It's about finding moments of connection in the everyday—in the beauty of nature, in acts of kindness, in the stillness of meditation. As I continue on this path, my spiritual practice has become a source of strength and comfort, guiding me through life's joys and challenges. It has taught me to approach the world with compassion, to seek the Divine in all things, and to trust in the unfolding journey of the soul.

From the church pews of my Southern childhood to the sacred peaks of the Himalayas, my spiritual journey has been one of continuous evolution. It is a testament to the power of remaining open, curious, and committed to personal growth. As I look to the future, I am filled with gratitude for the path that has led me here, and excitement for the spiritual discoveries that lie ahead.

Lisa Kaley-Isley
PhD, E-RYT-500, C-IAYT, USA

NO STRUGGLE—SIMPLY A GUIDED QUEST FOR TRUTH

My spiritual quest began innocently in childhood, between the ages of six and nine, when I would go out to my front yard in Philadelphia at night. I would gaze at the stars and play with a fascinating yet frightening mental exercise—imagining nothingness. I would systematically make things disappear in my mind—the traffic, the city, everything—until I reached a vast empty space. Although it often scared me enough to run back inside, these early experiences with contemplating nothingness planted important seeds.

Growing up, I observed my parents' relationship challenges, which made me question why people couldn't simply be honest and clear with each other. During my regular flights from Philadelphia to summer camp in Maine, I began having profound experiences of pure presence awareness. Once, while flying, I had a vivid memory of being on the plane the previous year, and time seemed to collapse into a single moment of consciousness. These experiences led me to believe there must be deeper answers in humanity's accumulated wisdom traditions.

Although my parents weren't particularly religious, we belonged to a conservative Jewish synagogue. While I enjoyed the chanting, I didn't feel deeply connected to the tradition. In college, my spiritual path took an unexpected turn when I enrolled in a Hindu studies course and discovered Patanjali's teachings. I took yoga as a physical education requirement, which led to studying Buddhism the following semester. My yoga teacher had studied with Krishnamacharya, which eventually led me to India.

In India, I studied *Shivite Siddhanta*, a South Indian tantric tradition, and had the privilege of private tutorials with a mystic scholar who chaired the Madras University Religious Studies Department. When my parents moved to Maui after my high school graduation, I became deeply involved with Tibetan Buddhism, serving on the board of the Maui Dharma Society for 20 years. In graduate school, I studied under Raimundo Panikkar, a Catholic priest who was also a Sanskrit scholar and authority on the *Vedas*.

My approach has always been practical, using yoga as a scientific method of self-investigation leading to self-realization. Unlike many who come to spiritual practice due to suffering, my journey was initiated by a deep faith and passionate curiosity. As a young religious studies student, I had the profound conviction that all spiritual traditions must be essentially true, even when they seemed contradictory. I believed that apparent paradoxes simply meant I needed to deepen my understanding.

Life presented various challenges that tested and strengthened my practice—marriage, divorce, my infant son's surgery, and, most significantly, my own health crisis. In 2004, I was diagnosed with a brain tumor requiring multiple surgeries. This experience profoundly deepened my understanding of yoga's true purpose, which my teacher had told me at age 19 was preparation for death. Through three major brain surgeries between 2004 and 2009, my decades of yoga practice proved invaluable.

The neurosurgeon was amazed at my psychological resilience, noting that many patients face severe emotional crises in similar situations. My intimate knowledge of my body through yoga practice had allowed me to detect subtle changes early, likely saving my life. Although I wouldn't wish such an experience on anyone, it accelerated my spiritual growth and transformed intellectual understanding into experiential wisdom.

My teacher once told me I was a "brusta"—one who had been on this spiritual journey in a past life but who hadn't completed it. This resonated deeply with my sense of having a living relationship with the tradition, enhanced through years of chanting and practice. Each challenge and suffering have served to deepen my understanding and transform it into wisdom.

I've been blessed to study with remarkable teachers from various traditions, fulfilling what a Vatican astrologer once told me about my chart, indicating connections with world teachers. While my experiential knowledge increasingly matches my intellectual understanding, I remain humble about the most elevated teachings. I see myself as still on the journey, experiencing ongoing maturation and deepening of wisdom.

In my work with others, I feel deeply guided. When working with individuals, I maintain focused periods of complete dedication to their process, allowing inner practices to emerge naturally rather than from intellectual planning. The meditations and teachings often come as direct transmissions rather than mental constructions.

The greatest gift of yoga has been understanding my multidimensional nature and learning to adapt these ancient tools to support my growth. I've come to recognize that my true identity lies beyond the visible—in the unchanging source of pure awareness. Yoga has helped me manage everything, from physical ailments to emotional challenges, while establishing values and priorities aligned with my deeper purpose (*svadharma*).

Today, I understand spirituality as simply reality itself—the recognition that life is a profound mystery. We do our best to understand what we can while remaining open to the unknown, acknowledging that we're not ultimately in control. This perspective has shaped my approach to teaching and sharing yoga therapy, emphasizing the importance of personal practice and respect for authentic traditions while maintaining the ability to meet each person where they are.

Although I haven't overcome all fear of death, I try to live each day as if my choices could be my last, seeking to live as fully as possible. My journey continues to unfold, guided by the wisdom of tradition and the direct experience of practice, always remembering that the deepest truths of yoga must be lived to be truly understood.

Gary Kraftsow
MA, E-RYT-500, C-IAYT, Founder/Director of
American Viniyoga Institute, LC, USA

FROM DEPRESSION TO DIVINE CONSCIOUSNESS

I never imagined that depression would be the catalyst for my spiritual awakening. Growing up in Ohio without any religious foundation—my mother's difficult experience with Catholicism had led her to let me choose my own path—I found myself in college, grappling with undiagnosed depression that would unexpectedly open doors to something greater.

My earliest connection to what would become my life's path began innocently enough, watching Lilian Folan's yoga classes on PBS in the 1970s. As a young child of four or five, I would mimic her graceful movements, drawn to the beauty and flow of the practice. Little did I know then how profoundly yoga would shape my life.

The pivotal moment came when I was 21, power walking along the river. Without warning, everything I knew about being "Stephanie" dissolved. The boundaries between my body and the world around me—the brick buildings, the highway, the trees, the sky—simply vanished. For about 15 minutes, there was a boundless experience as pure consciousness, everywhere and nowhere at once. When the feeling of separation, or existing within my body, returned, everything felt mechanical, and there was a metallic taste in my mouth. Although overwhelming, it wasn't frightening; instead, it filled me with wonder and tears.

This experience sparked an intense search for understanding. Like many seekers, I experimented with hallucinogens—LSD and magic mushrooms—trying to recreate that state of consciousness. Looking back, I see how I was playing with the ego's need for control versus the pure flow that emerged when it surrendered. Thankfully, my journey also led me to more grounded practices. I discovered *Kripalu Yoga* through a remarkable teacher who was both a nurse and a disciple of Amrit Desai. She recognized my devotion to *sadhana*, even performing a ceremony to certify me as a true yogini.

Moving to Chicago opened new doors. Under Per Erez's guidance, I experienced *yoga nidra* for the first time, which resonated deeply with my earlier spiritual awakening. Although I was still working through personal challenges—anxiety, depression, and what I'd call neurotic tendencies—these practices began to ground me.

The mystical experiences continued to unfold in everyday moments. Once, while working as a hospice social worker, I was driving down the highway when that same dissolution of self occurred. Consciousness expanded beyond my body, embracing the cars around me, Lake Michigan, the field, everything. The perfection and acceptance of that moment brought me to tears—tears of recognition of the vast heart of being. I pulled over, awed by the experience, and called a Buddhist chaplain who helped me ground myself before continuing my workday.

These experiences began happening more frequently. Sometimes walls would undulate, or the ground beneath my feet would shift. Rather than fear these phenomena, I learned to integrate them into my daily life, balancing them with my work as a social worker and my personal relationships. Even at my wedding celebration I experienced a profound moment where I could see the essential nature shining through everyone's eyes, as if all were already awakened.

Meeting Richard Miller was like coming home. For the first time, someone could articulate what I had experienced all those years ago. He helped me understand these experiences within a broader context, and provided practices to help my system become more sensitive to the subtle realms of consciousness. Under his guidance, I began to understand that these weren't just isolated mystical experiences but part of a deeper awakening process.

The impact on my professional life was profound. My approach to therapy and yoga teaching transformed completely. Instead of working from a "fixing" mindset, I began recognizing the inherent wholeness in everyone I worked with. Whether someone came to me for anxiety, grief, depression, or life transitions, my role became about creating space for them to discover their own essential nature, which brought new insights and possibilities as they were meeting life's challenges.

The most precious gift yoga has given me is the recognition of the Self with a capital "S"—the understanding that goes beyond our stories to touch the essence of the human condition. It's provided a comprehensive framework for attuning to our deepest nature, moving from the physical practices of *asana* through the subtleties of *pranayama*, meditation, and ultimately to the shore of the Infinite.

Now, when I sit with clients, there's a different quality of presence—a deeper listening, an open-hearted welcoming that creates space for others to ease into their own exploration. This isn't about imposing spiritual concepts but about meeting people where they are. The traditional therapeutic tools are still there—assessment, goal-setting, practical interventions—but they're held within a larger context of fundamental wholeness.

After 33 years since that first awakening, I've learned that while the mind still functions, it serves a different purpose. Rather than mind or ego being the orienting principle of living, an interconnected wholeness is the source. The essence is always here, waiting to be recognized. The journey continues to unfold, revealing new depths of understanding and presence with each passing day.

To young yoga teachers and therapists, I offer this advice: Start with yourself. Pay attention to what's calling you. Don't rush past your own experience in search of knowledge from books or others. Our presence is what makes all the difference—when we come from a place of genuine openness and recognition of wholeness, rather than from a need to fix or change, we create space for profound transformation in the client.

The path of yoga has shown me that awakening isn't just about transcendent experiences or achieving particular states of consciousness; it's about recognizing the vast essence of being that's always present, always whole, always complete, and embodying this truth, moment to moment. Whether I'm leading a meditation, conducting a therapy session, or simply moving through my daily life, this understanding continues to deepen and evolve, informing every aspect of my being and my work in the world.

Stephanie Lopez
LISW-S, C-IAYT, Senior Advisor of Philosophy & Learning,
iRest Institute, USA

CHAPTER 11

Spirituality in Action

In the tapestry of human experience, few threads are as vibrant and transformative as those woven by spiritual awakening. The following six stories weave together themes of trauma, healing, self-discovery, and interconnectedness, offering a deeply personal yet universally resonant perspective on spiritual growth.

ROOTS OF THE SPIRIT: THROUGH TRAUMA AND HEALING

My story begins on a small island, where, as a young girl, I spent my summers in solitude, embracing the quiet companionship of blueberry bushes and ancient rocks. It was here, in this secluded paradise, that I first felt the stirrings of something greater than myself—a connection to the depth of my soul and the universe—that transcended the physical world around me.

Little did I know then that this early communion with nature would become my anchor through the storms of life that lay ahead. When I was 22, my world shattered with the sudden death of my younger brother in a motorcycle accident. It was a pivotal moment, one that forced me to confront the harsh reality of impermanence and loss. In the depths of my grief, I found myself instinctively turning to the lessons the natural world had taught me—the art of letting go, of flowing with the cycles of life and death.

Years passed, and I found myself pregnant with my fourth child, brimming with the joy and anticipation that only an expectant mother can know. But fate had other plans. Two weeks before my due date, my son Brody was stillborn, the umbilical cord knotted in a cruel twist of destiny. In that moment, as I held his lifeless body in my arms, I felt as though I had given birth to death itself.

It was in these darkest of hours that I first turned to yoga, not just as a physical practice, but as a spiritual seatbelt. The philosophy and tools of yoga became my guiding light, helping me navigate the treacherous waters of grief and loss. I clung to the belief that Brody's spirit would return when the time was right, and miraculously, just months later, I conceived again. When my daughter Tessa was born, I felt in my heart that Brody's essence had found its way back to me.

This belief, this story I tell myself, has been my refuge. It's not about intellectual reasoning; it's about finding a narrative that keeps me tethered to hope and purpose when the world seems intent on pulling me under. Yoga taught me to breathe through the pain, to find stillness in the chaos, and to connect with something greater than my individual suffering.

But life wasn't done testing my resilience. Just as the world was emerging from the grips of the Covid-19 pandemic, my daughter Tessa—the very child I believed carried Brody's spirit—was diagnosed with an aggressive form of leukemia at the age of 18. For nine grueling months, we lived in and out of hospitals, facing each new challenge with the full scope of tools yoga had given me.

During those long days and longer nights, I would take morning baths, using the time to meditate and repeat my mantra: "This is traumatic, *and* I will be okay. She will be okay." I drew upon every aspect of yoga philosophy—the *kleshas*, the *koshas*, the *doshas*—to keep myself grounded and present.

It wasn't just about the physical practice, which I did when I could, sometimes in those morning baths. Although these did release tensions of the body created by emotions living in my body, it was all about embracing the release of those emotions and breathing through the fear. It allowed me to stay connected to that inner spark of divinity, which I believe resides in all of us, waiting for us to return to it to stabilize us when our world spins.

As I watched my daughter practice her own gentle form of yoga during her recovery, I witnessed firsthand the power of this ancient practice to heal not just the body, but also the spirit. It was a profound reminder that spirituality isn't about adhering to rigid doctrines or complex rituals; it's about finding what resonates with your soul, and using it as a seatbelt when the currents of life threaten to sweep you away.

Throughout these trials, I've come to understand that spirituality is deeply personal. For some, it's found in the hallowed halls of churches or temples. For others, like myself, it's in the quiet embrace of a forest or the gentle lapping of waves on a lakeshore. What matters is not the form it takes, but the comfort and strength it provides.

My role as a yoga teacher and therapist is not to impose my beliefs on others, but to help my students uncover their own connection to something greater than themselves. I'm careful with how I introduce the concept of spirituality. I know that for some the word itself can be off-putting, laden with negative associations or past traumas. Instead, I focus on the universal experiences that connect us all—the awe we feel when witnessing a beautiful sunset or the peace that descends during a moment of true stillness.

As I've navigated my own path through joy and sorrow, I've learned that life rarely unfolds according to our carefully laid plans. I've abandoned the notion of trying to control my destiny and instead embraced the metaphor of a canoe journey. I put my canoe in the water, get in, and start paddling, but I don't try to dictate where the current will take me. This approach has led me to unexpected places, including the development of my yoga therapy practice—a calling that emerged from a series of seemingly random encounters and heartbreaks.

Looking back, I can see how each challenge, each loss, has shaped me and deepened my spiritual practice. The death of my brother, taught me by my father's example of putting healing over bitterness after my brother's death, taught me the power of personal choice. The loss of my son Brody showed me the profound connection between birth and death. My father's passing reinforced the importance of breathing through life's difficulties without questioning every twist and turn.

As I continue on this journey, I'm constantly reminded that spirituality isn't about having all the answers; it's about being comfortable with the questions, with the mystery of existence. It's about finding peace in the connection to something greater than ourselves, whether we call it God, the universe, or simply the energy that binds all living things.

My experiences have taught me that while suffering is an inevitable part of life, we have the power to choose how we respond to it. By staying connected to our inner spirit, by breathing through the pain, and by trusting in the flow of life, we can find strength and purpose, even in our darkest hours.

Helene Couvrette
C-IAYT, E-RYT-500, Yoga Educator, Founder/President
H~OM Yoga School, Cofounder/President MISTY (Montreal
International Symposium on Therapeutic Yoga), Canada

A SELF-DISCOVERY

As I sit down to write this chapter of my life, I'm struck by the profound journey that has led me to where I am today. My name is Richard Miller, and my path to self-realization began before I could even form coherent thoughts.

I remember vividly, at the tender age of two, the moment when the world suddenly materialized around me. My sister, the room, the bed, the windows—all these concepts that hadn't existed before suddenly came into being. It was as if a veil had been lifted, and with it came the first inkling of separation. This feeling that something wasn't quite right would follow me for years to come.

As a teenager, lying under the Florida night sky, I had my first taste of unity with the universe. Pondering the limits of existence, I imagined jumping over cosmic walls until everything dissolved, and I was left with a profound sense of peace and oneness with everything. But, like many adolescents, I couldn't hold onto this feeling, and the nagging sense of something not right persisted.

It wasn't until I was 22, taking my first yoga class in San Francisco, that I experienced the oneness again. The simple *yoga nidra* practice left me feeling whole, free from the depression that had become my constant companion. This experience planted a seed, one that would grow into a lifelong pursuit of understanding and embodying this state of being.

My journey led me through various spiritual and psychological paths. I studied with a woman who blended Buddhist, yoga and Western psychological approaches. I delved into Taoism and Chinese medicine, considered becoming a Jesuit priest, and ultimately found my way to a PhD in Clinical Psychology.

But it was my encounter with Jean Klein, my spiritual teacher, that truly deepened my practice. Under his guidance, I had more and more glimpses of my true nature. Then, one early morning in 1996, it happened. There were no fireworks, no grand epiphany—just a gentle recognition of my essential self. It was as if a switch had been flipped and I couldn't turn it off.

This recognition brought with it a pervasive sense of joy and well-being that has remained constant, even in the face of grief, pain, and challenging circumstances. It's not that I don't experience these difficult emotions—I do. But underlying it all is an unshakeable peace, a connection to the essence of being that permeates every experience.

As a psychotherapist, I've had the privilege of helping others navigate their own journeys. I've learned that by creating a space for people to glimpse their essential nature, even for a moment, we can spark profound change. I've seen chronic pain disappear, trauma heal, and lives transform through the practices of yoga and mindfulness.

But I've also come to understand that this work isn't about fixing or changing ourselves; it's about peeling away the layers of conditioning, the self-images we've accumulated over a lifetime. As my early mentor, Laura, advised me: "Look in the mirror until you've peeled away all your self-images and you realize that you'll never see yourself. The seer can't see itself because it's not an object."

This process of shedding our constructed identities can be terrifying at times. As my old identity of Richard began to dissemble, I experienced moments of sheer terror. But there was always an underlying curiosity, a willingness to lean into the discomfort and say, "Bring it on!"

I've come to see that enlightenment doesn't mean the absence of preferences or the elimination of our basic human responses. Our nervous systems are still wired to assess for danger, to have likes and dislikes. The difference is in how we relate to these experiences. We can observe them without getting caught up in them, understanding them as part of our human experience without being defined by them.

As I reflect on my journey, I'm filled with gratitude for the gift of yoga and the path of inquiry it has opened up for me. It's shown me that no amount of physical prowess or breath control can make me "better"—that the state of consciousness we seek is independent of any doing. And yet, for this body and mind, the teachings of yoga were the vehicle that brought me home to myself.

I continue to be amazed by the mystery of it all. How is it that some of us stumble into profound spiritual realization while others don't? Why did I meet the exact people I needed to meet at the exact right times? Life unfolds in its own inscrutable way, and our job is simply to show up, to do the work we're called to do, and to trust in the process.

To those on their own path of self-discovery, I offer this advice: Be willing to look deeply at yourself, to peel away the layers of conditioning and self-image. Set your personality free and discover what remains when all pretense falls away. And above all, cultivate a sense of curiosity and openness to whatever arises.

In the end, this journey isn't about becoming something other than what we are. It's about recognizing our true nature, which has been here all along. It's about falling in love with ourselves and with life itself, in all its messy, beautiful complexity. And it's about sharing that love with others, creating moments of sacred connection in the most unexpected places—even in line for tacos at a farmer's market.

As I continue to teach and learn, to meet each moment with openness and love, I'm continually reminded of the beauty, preciousness, and mystery of this human experience. We are all on this journey together, each in our own way, finding our path back to the essence of who we truly are.

Richard Miller
PhD, F-IAYT, E-RYT-500, Founder of iRest, USA

AWAKENING: FROM PETROCHEMICALS TOWARDS ENLIGHTENMENT

As I reflect on my transformative journey of spiritual awakening, I'm transported back to when I was just 20 years old. At that time, my focus, like many my age, was solely on saving money to attend university and pursue a career in engineering. I was working in the petrochemical industry, specifically in Texaco's lab research, and I felt incredibly excited about my future academic prospects.

Almost overnight, a profound and inexplicable feeling of depression descended upon me. It was as if a thief had crept into my consciousness, stealing away my certainty and leaving me with a deep sense of unease. Suddenly, the path I had been so sure of—the pursuit of a degree, diploma, title, and position—seemed hollow and unfulfilling.

This depression that enveloped me brought with it startling realizations: I couldn't control my thoughts, I didn't truly know love, and I was completely lost when it came to understanding my own identity and purpose in life. As it was, this shift coincided with a significant astrological period in my life. The planetary alignments were changing, heralding a transformation in my very being.

Life's existential questions consumed me. I found myself constantly pondering: Who am I really? Where did I come from? Where am I going? The intensity of these thoughts was overwhelming, keeping me in a state of confusion and emotional turmoil.

Seeking answers, I turned to metaphysics, a subject that had fascinated me since I was 15 or 16 years old. I devoured books on the subject, reading biographies of individuals who seemed to have found something profound in their spiritual quests. With my scientific background, I approached spirituality methodically, wanting a deeper experience, but through testing, experimentation, and exploration.

In my search, I realized what I truly needed was a genuine master—someone who had walked the spiritual path and who could guide me based on their own experiences. This realization became my driving force, and for an entire year, I dedicated myself to seeking out spiritual groups and researching different paths.

I even changed my job, moving from the petrochemical industry to teaching, all while saving money for what I knew would be a transformative journey to India. At age 21, with no plans of looking back, I embarked on my quest to find true masters in the spiritual heartland of the East.

My journey led me to several enlightening encounters, but it was at Swami

Muktananda's ashram that my life truly changed. Within days of arriving, I experienced an awakening of *kundalini* energy that was both profound and unmistakable. This energy took control of my body, moving me in mystical dances, filling my heart with an indescribable sense of love and connection.

I began to feel as though God was awakening within me. The energy was purely benevolent, and I found myself responding to music and chanting in ways I never had before. My voice would rise from within, and I felt a power greater than my physical body or mind guiding my actions.

Reading about *kundalini* and *shaktipat* in the ashram's library, I began to make sense of these new experiences I was having. I realized that what I was going through was a profound spiritual awakening (known as *shaktipat*), influenced by the presence of a true master—Baba Muktananda—even though he was not physically present in the ashram during that time.

For weeks, I immersed myself in ashram life. I found joy in simple activities—working in the gardens, helping in the kitchen, tending to the cows. Everything I did felt infused with this new, benevolent presence. I wasn't scared of these experiences because they brought with them a sense of freedom, love, and happiness.

My relationship with the world around me transformed. I felt a deep connection to a universal power, which was comforting and exhilarating. This energy became my guru, guiding me and improving every aspect of my being—my body felt healthier, my mind more at peace, and my heart more open to love and compassion.

After leaving the ashram, I traveled through India, visiting sacred places and finding that this energy would resurface in these spiritual environments. I learned to maintain this connection through spiritual disciplines like chanting and meditation.

Returning home after four transformative months in India, I was a changed person. I resumed teaching, but with a newfound joy and connection to my students and colleagues. The depression that had plagued me was gone, replaced by a deep sense of purpose and contentment.

Two years later, I returned to Baba Muktananda's ashram for teacher training. It was during this time that I had my first physical encounter with Baba. Initially, I felt strangely alienated from his physical form, having focused so long on the internal energy. But as I closed my eyes and reconnected with that inner power, I realized that Baba was operating from the same energy I had experienced. This insight transformed my understanding of who a guru truly is.

Before leaving the ashram, I had a brief but profound interaction with Baba.

It is then that he gifted me my spiritual name, Vasudeva, and endowed a blessing with his walking stick as I bowed reverently to him. I felt a complete oneness with this being in that moment.

On my return home, I established a meditation center and continued my spiritual practice. Seven months later brought me to an intense 40-day period of transformation. This energy, which had been concentrated in my brow, shifted to my crown *chakra*, bringing with it an overwhelming feeling of complete freedom. I felt completely unburdened, transcending the limitations of my human form to now experiencing being an instrument of a far greater power.

This experience deepened my connection to the universe. I found myself centered in what felt like the heart of the cosmos, with access to infinite wisdom and peace. My intuition sharpened, and I developed the ability to feel and understand our subtle energy anatomy through the *chakras*.

This gift became the foundation of my work as a teacher, yoga therapist, and healer. I learned to guide people through meditation, helping them clear their *chakras* and lift out of darkness. My approach to therapy is holistic, emphasizing the importance of self-work for any healer or therapist.

Looking back on my journey, I'm grateful for the wisdom that has allowed me to navigate this path. To those on a similar journey, I emphasize the importance of self-discovery and self-empowerment. True healing comes not just from external treatments, but also from helping people understand their own spiritual nature and innate healing powers.

Sri Vasudeva
International Spiritual Teacher, Trinidad & Tobago

BEYOND THE VEIL: LIFE, DEATH, AND YOGA

I am awestruck by the profound experiences that can shape our understanding of life, death, and the human spirit. One story, which occurred some five decades ago, continues to define my existence and leads me onward.

When I was just 10 years old, on a seemingly ordinary day, I attempted to cross a rushing river with my father and brother. The three of us held hands. The water was cold, and rushed around us. I felt a sense of exhilaration and freedom. In a split second, everything changed when I slipped on a rock. Suddenly, an overwhelming sense of fear took over as I fought for my life. My father lifted both my brother and me above the water for air, until there came a moment when I wasn't lifted up and I knew—I was drowning.

In less than a blink of an eye, I was transported to another world—a realm beyond physical reality. A place not subject to time. How do you describe the indescribable? The emotions I felt were unlike anything I had ever experienced. A state of all-encompassing peace, a feeling of complete acceptance and understanding.

In this otherworldly place, I encountered what I can only describe as a spirit guide. The communication between us was telepathic, a pure exchange of consciousness. This being knew me instantly, in a way that transcended any earthly relationship. There was no judgment, only recognition and acceptance. And pure love.

In this joyous, expansive state, I felt a magnetic pull urging me to continue onward, toward what I can only describe as "the Presence." But then came a pivotal moment. The spirit guide asked if I wanted to continue. In my mind, I couldn't fathom why anyone would choose to return to the earthly realm fraught with suffering. Yet, in an instant, with the thought of my mother, I was returned to the river, returned to fighting for my life.

I returned with a profound understanding that life has a valuable purpose. At 10 years old, I couldn't fully grasp what that meant, but I knew deep in my soul that not just my life, but all life, has significance.

This near-death experience (NDE) was the most profound experience of my life, and has shaped every aspect of it, instilling a deep sense of empathy, a connection to others that goes beyond the superficial. I've come to realize that this heightened empathy is common among those who've crossed over and returned. We come back changed, with a different perspective on life and death, and a deep knowing of our ephemeral nature in this world.

For years, I kept this experience to myself, feeling like an oddity—a "freak." It wasn't until I was 20 that I first spoke about it with my father, only to discover that he, too, had had an NDE. This revelation opened the floodgates. I began to explore and study other accounts, finding solace in the shared experiences of others and our ability to more easily permeate the membrane that separates this world from the afterlife, like muscle memory.

The first yoga class I attended was in a gym when I was in my early 30s. While I can't recall the teacher's face or name, I vividly remember how the practice made me feel: similar to the place beyond the river. Initially, I incorporated yoga into my cardio routine. It wasn't until an injury led me to a physical therapist who prescribed yoga postures that I realized the richness of yoga. The healing I experienced through *asana* was transformative, and I knew instinctively that I had to practice more often and learn more about yoga, and that I wanted to...had to...share it.

Despite my lack of formal training, I began teaching on the church lawn. I started with just one student who became a dear friend and promoter of the free classes, which included meditation and guided imagery. My practice and teaching style evolved, and students often described the classes as "spiritual" and "holding sacred space." Some asked where I had completed my teacher training. I could have said *in the place beyond the river.*

I delved deeper into yoga through formal certification, which is where I first learned of yoga therapy. It resonated deeply with my experiences and desires to introduce others to the healing qualities of the ancient practice. Studying yoga therapy has led me to where I am today, using yoga as a tool for healing and connection in both inpatient and outpatient settings.

My NDE not only shaped my spiritual path but also enhanced my intuitive abilities. I've experienced dream-state communications and received messages from the dead and unborn. These experiences have reinforced my belief in the permeable nature of the veil between life and death.

In my daily life and work, I strive to maintain a connection to that otherworldly realm. Through meditation, mantras, and my yoga practice, especially *yoga nidra*, I feel closer to that permeable membrane separating our world from the next. This connection guides my interactions with patients/clients, allowing me to offer support and healing in ways that go beyond the physical.

As I reflect on my journey, I'm filled with gratitude for the experiences that have shaped me. The NDE that could have ended my life instead gives it profound meaning and purpose. It teaches me about the power of love, the importance of empathy, and the interconnectedness of all beings. As we say, the issue can become the portal, the gateway to change. And so, the NDE has been exactly that.

Each of us has the ability to tap into something greater than ourselves. When we practice, we are not importing anything new. Instead, we are returning to the inner knowing that is timeless and true. Whether through meditation, yoga, or simply being open to the universe's guidance, we can access to wisdom and love that transcends our everyday existence.

As I continue to teach, and explore the depths of human consciousness, I carry with me the lessons learned from my brush with death. I show up, I work, I meditate, I have a practice, but I'm not acting alone. The guidance comes in a feeling and a knowing of "the Voice." The density of "Presence" yet expansiveness! It comes from outside and it's inside me.

My story is just one of many, a testament to the extraordinary experiences that shape our lives and the unseen forces that guide us. As you read these words, I invite you to reflect on your own journey, to be open to the mysteries of the universe, and to embrace the love and purpose that exists within each of us.

Julie Rowland
C-IAYT, Certified Yoga Therapist, UCLA Health Integrative
Medicine Collaborative, Ornish Lifestyle Medicine, Loyola
Marymount University, Yoga Therapy Mentor, USA

YOGA, GRIEF, AND SPIRITUAL AWAKENING

My journey through yoga began in my childhood, with my grandmother as my first teacher, introducing me to *asana*, *pranayama*, and meditation. Little did I know then how profoundly these early lessons would shape my life.

The AIDS epidemic of the 1980s and 1990s became a crucible for my practice. Overwhelmed by grief, I found myself drawn back to yoga, stumbling into a class that echoed my grandmother's teachings. This "divine coincidence" reconnected me with the *Integral Yoga* lineage of Swami Satchidananda, setting the stage for a deeper exploration of yoga's spiritual dimensions.

During those early days, I was an AIDS activist, and I spent many years organizing and going to demonstrations, and getting arrested over and over again. I was getting burned out, and I finally realized that I could share yoga with my community as a way to serve and support them. I ended up graduating from yoga teacher training in 1995, and immediately started teaching classes for people with HIV and AIDS in a local hospital in the Castro district in San Francisco.

I remember one very special experience that happened after a few years of teaching there. The class was made up of gay men with HIV and AIDS. It was a beautiful community that we formed in the midst of such devastation. One day, we were sitting in a circle meditating at the end of class, and to my surprise, as I opened my eyes, I saw a golden chord connecting us all, from the top of our heads. It was like this circle of golden light that was holding us together. It really blew my mind. In fact, I had a really hard time coming out of that meditation to end class!

Illness and death has always motivated my practice. Perhaps it's a universal motivator for spiritual practice? But with the AIDS epidemic, it was just so much death, and for me, it was so much to handle at such a young age. In those days AIDS was not treatable.

My best friend Kurt, who died of AIDS in 1995, really encouraged me to practice and teach yoga. In particular, he was obsessed with the concept of nonattachment. He would make a list of his attachments every day and he would often read the list to me. He would get particularly excited if he had taken something off his list—like he had successfully let it go, or said goodbye to it. I didn't quite understand at the time what that meant, but looking back, I see that he was consciously dying.

He read me the list, and it had his boyfriend, his dog, his apartment, and me on it. We were the top four! I was all excited that I had made the top four. He said he was challenged by these four things, and he wasn't able to let them go. One day I went to see him in the hospital, and he was so excited. He said, "Oh, I got my list down to two things—Randy [his boyfriend] and Buddy [his dog]." I was confused. So I asked him, "Wait, that's a good thing? I'm off the list?" So he explained, "Yes, you're my dear spiritual friend, and we'll always be together because I love you." It was very sweet, but I still didn't quite understand.

Then a few weeks later, when he died, I remembered what he had said, and it gave me solace. I could feel that he was still with me. In fact, we had a little funeral, just a few of us gathered, and I felt much lighter than I had expected. I thought, "Oh, I think that's what he meant. He let me go, and consciously said goodbye to me." It was a generous gift that actually made it easier for me to let go as well.

I don't think our relationship with someone ends when they die. It just changes the form of the relationship. I try to focus on the yoga teachings that explain that we're spiritual beings, *purusha*, and that the body and mind, *prakriti*, are temporary and constantly changing, and they eventually die. The practice is to recognize that their heart, or the love they shared with you, is still there. It's never changed and can never change. Of course, it's a practice, and grief is a tricky emotion, but yoga helps through the practice of connecting to the eternal.

These profound experiences with death, community, and spirituality gave birth to my vision for Accessible Yoga. My mission became clear: to make the deeper aspects of yoga available to all, regardless of physical ability, background, or life circumstance. I recognized that the true challenge in making yoga accessible wasn't just about adapting physical postures, but about conveying the essential spiritual teachings in an understandable and relatable way.

My path wasn't without its challenges. The revelation of sexual abuse within my spiritual lineage forced me to confront difficult truths about authority and personal agency in spiritual practice. This experience, although painful, reinforced my belief in the importance of empowering individuals to be their own gurus, and to find wisdom within themselves and the teachings rather than relying solely on external figures.

As a yoga therapist and teacher, I've come to emphasize the importance of intuition. I view it as a way to transcend the limitations of the ego and connect with a deeper wisdom. My approach involves staying open and responsive to the needs of the moment, often relying on feelings and spontaneous insights that arise during interactions with clients.

For those entering the field of yoga therapy, I offer two key pieces of advice. First, focus on empowering the client, recognizing that the therapist doesn't need to have all the answers, but rather should create a space for the client's own wisdom to emerge. Second, maintain a strong personal practice (*sadhana*), as this is the foundation for being present and intuitive with clients. Having a strong ethical structure for our teaching, or, to put it simply, having strong boundaries, is the other essential part about serving as a yoga teacher or therapist.

Drawing from my experiences as a gay man during the AIDS crisis, I've come to recognize the spiritual potential in being an outsider. I believe that those who feel different or marginalized often have an intuitive grasp of spiritual concepts that others must work to understand. This perspective informs my work with Accessible Yoga, celebrating diversity as a pathway to deeper spiritual insight.

As I continue to write and teach, I'm reminded that in our differences and challenges we often find our greatest teachers and our deepest connections to the universal truths that yoga seeks to illuminate. This journey has shown me the transformative power of yoga, not just as a physical practice, but as a comprehensive approach to life, death, and everything in between.

Jivana Heyman
C-IAYT, E-RYT-500, Director, Accessible Yoga, USA

THE MODERN YOGI: BRIDGING TRADITION AND SCIENCE

In the realm of yoga therapy, few individuals embody the seamless integration of ancient wisdom and modern science quite like Yogacharya Dr. Ananda Balayogi Bhavanani. Born into a lineage of yoga masters and raised in an ashram, yet educated as a medical doctor, Bhavanani's life story offers profound insights into the spiritual dimensions of yoga therapy and its potential to transform both practitioner and patient.

Bhavanani's journey begins with an extraordinary childhood. Born to a half-Indian, half-Irish father and an American mother, he was immersed in a world where spirituality permeated every aspect of daily life. In the ashram, cooking, teaching, and even mundane tasks were infused with spiritual significance. This early exposure shaped his worldview, instilling in him the understanding that spirituality was not separate from everyday existence, but integral to it.

The young Bhavanani witnessed firsthand the power of inclusivity and unity. The ashram welcomed children from all backgrounds, transcending the rigid caste divisions prevalent in Indian society. This experience of oneness with diverse individuals became a cornerstone of Bhavanani's spiritual philosophy, emphasizing the celebration of diversity within unity.

Perhaps the most profound spiritual experiences of Bhavanani's youth occurred during ceremonies honoring the gurus of his tradition. He recalls moments of transcendence where the vibrations of chanting seemed to transport him to other planes of existence. These experiences forged a deep, soul-to-soul connection with the gurus, which continues to guide him to this day.

This connection manifests as an inner voice, a source of clarity and guidance that Bhavanani has learned to trust implicitly. It is this inner wisdom, emanating from what yoga philosophy calls the *anandamaya kosha* (the bliss sheath), that he believes is crucial for yoga therapists to access and embody in their work.

Bhavanani's entry into the world of modern medicine presented a stark contrast to his upbringing. The reverence and gratitude he felt towards the human body, even in dissection, was at odds with the detached, sometimes disrespectful attitudes of his peers. This experience highlighted the need to bridge the gap between the spiritual approach of yoga and the scientific rigor of modern medicine.

As Bhavanani ventured into the field of yoga therapy, he encountered a community often more focused on techniques than on the transformative power of the therapist–client relationship. He emphasizes that yoga therapy is not merely about prescribing specific *asanas* or *pranayamas* for particular conditions; instead, it is about facilitating a holistic healing process that addresses the whole person.

Bhavanani distinguishes between curing (eradicating pathology) and healing (restoring wholeness). While modern medicine excels at curing, yoga therapy offers the potential for deep healing by reconnecting individuals with their sense of self and purpose.

Central to Bhavanani's philosophy is the concept of *sadhana*, the consistent practice and living of yoga principles. He argues that without a lived experience of yoga, a therapist cannot be authentic, and without authenticity, transformation cannot occur. This *sadhana* extends beyond formal practice on the mat to encompass every moment of life.

Through dedicated *sadhana*, yoga therapists undergo their own transformation and transcendence. This lived experience becomes the wellspring from which they can truly help others, embodying the teachings in a way that clients can sense and begin to emulate.

Bhavanani advocates for a balanced approach that honors both the living tradition of yoga and the insights gained through scientific research. He cautions against relying solely on standardized protocols, emphasizing the need for intuition and adaptability in addressing each client's unique needs. This balance requires yoga therapists to continually engage with both traditional teachings and emerging scientific understanding. It's a dynamic process of integration, where lived experience serves as the crucible in which tradition and science are alchemized into effective, personalized therapy.

At the heart of Bhavanani's approach is recognizing the spiritual nature of the therapeutic relationship. He emphasizes the importance of respecting each client's dignity and individuality, creating a space where they feel valued and cared for. This soul-to-soul connection allows clients to experience the transformative power of yoga on a deep level.

Bhavanani argues that the therapist cannot be separate from the therapy. By accessing their own *anandamaya kosha*, therapists create a resonance that allows clients to connect with their own inner wisdom and potential for healing.

Bhavanani often expresses concern about the trend in modern yoga therapy to adopt models from other therapeutic disciplines without fully embracing yoga's unique spiritual perspective. He cautions against the over-medicalization of yoga therapy, which risks losing the heart and soul of the practice. While he supports the integration of yoga into medical education, Bhavanani stresses that becoming a yoga therapist requires more than just adding yoga techniques to existing medical knowledge. It demands a paradigm shift from a disease-focused approach to a holistic, salutogenic model that emphasizes health and well-being.

Despite his privileged background in yoga, Bhavanani has dedicated his life to making these teachings accessible to all. He strives to present yoga therapy in pragmatic, digestible ways that resonate with people from all walks of life. His journey of self-inquiry and continuous learning serves as an inspiration for aspiring yoga therapists.

In conclusion, Bhavanani's life and teachings offer a compelling vision for the future of yoga therapy. By bridging the spiritual wisdom of yoga with the insights of modern science, and by emphasizing the transformative power of authentic, lived experience, he points the way toward a more holistic and effective approach to healing. As yoga therapy continues to evolve, Bhavanani's emphasis on the spiritual dimension of this work serves as a vital reminder of its true potential to transform lives and promote deep, lasting healing.

As we navigate the complex landscape of modern healthcare and spiritual practice, voices like Bhavanani's are essential. They remind us of the profound potential of ancient wisdom when applied with understanding and authenticity in our modern world. They challenge us to expand our consciousness, to embody our highest principles, and to approach healing as a holistic, spiritual endeavor.

In the end, the journey of a yoga therapist, as Bhavanani describes it, is not so different from the spiritual journey we're all on—a journey of continuous growth, of expanding awareness, and of learning to embody our highest potential in service of others. It's a journey that requires both the grounding of tradition and the openness to new understanding, both the heart's wisdom and the head's discernment. And it's a journey that, ultimately, leads us to a deeper connection with ourselves, with others, and with the vast, interconnected web of life of which we're all a part.

(This story was written based on Lee Majewski's interview with Yogacharya Dr. Ananda Balayogi Bhavanani, Ashram Acharya, ICYER-Ananda Ashram, Madathipathi, Sri Kambaliswamy Madam, Chairman and Mentor Yoganjali Natyalayam, Director and Professor of Yoga Therapy, Institute of Salutogenesis and Complementary Medicine, Sri Balaji Vidyapeeth, Pondicherry, India)

Epilogue

As we come to the end of this book, I feel tremendous gratitude to all my friends – long term yoga practitioners – who so generously shared their life stories here. These stories are testaments to yoga not simply as a physical discipline or set of techniques, but as a living tradition – a bridge between ancient wisdom and contemporary needs.

We all feel deep appreciation of this ancient wisdom that offered each of us a road map for the expansion of consciousness, invited us to move beyond the confines of ego, reconnect with our bodies and emotions, and ultimately led us to experience the unity that underlies all existence. In doing so, yoga helped us to address our core spiritual needs identified throughout this book: the search for meaning, the longing for connection, and the desire for healing and wholeness.

My aim was to trace metamorphosis of spirituality from the decline of traditional religious affiliation to the rise of secular spirituality, from the scientific exploration of consciousness to the deeply personal stories of transformation. Hopefully this process reveals to the reader a profound truth: spirituality is neither a relic of the past nor the exclusive domain of any faith. Rather, it is an intrinsic dimension of human experience, endlessly adaptable, and essential for individual and collective flourishing. Science increasingly affirms what mystics have long known: that our well-being is intimately tied to our sense of purpose, our capacity for awe, and our ability to experience ourselves as part of something greater.

May this book bring the discussion on spirituality to our kitchen tables, to our family discussion not as part of any religion but as a way of being through yoga – a continual process of awakening, integrating, and embodying our highest values. In a world marked by rapid change, fragmentation, and existential uncertainty, yoga and the insights of secular spirituality offer not only solace but also a call to action: to live more consciously, to care more deeply, and to co-create communities rooted in empathy and purpose.

This path ahead is not one of perfection but of perpetual becoming, where every moment offers an opportunity to awaken – to shed the illusion of separateness and embrace the boundless potential of your true nature. Through yoga, one experiences spirituality not as a relic of the past but as a compass for the future. In a world grappling with loneliness, polarization, and ecological crisis, the cultivation of such spiritual awareness offers a path to healing – for individuals, communities, and perhaps our planet itself.

In the words of the *Bhagavad Gita* (6.5–6):

> Let one lift oneself by oneself; let one not degrade oneself. For the Self is one's own friend, and the Self is one's own enemy. To him who has conquered the Self by the Self, the Self is a friend. But to him who has not conquered the Self, the Self remains hostile.

The peace and happiness you seek is already within you. Let the yoga practice, your presence, and your compassion illuminate the path to your highest Self. The journey continues.

Namaste.

List of Interviewees

CHAPTER 7, BREAKING FREE
Leanne Davis, C-IAYT, Doctor of Acupuncture, Bachelor of Health Science (Acupuncture), Yoga Therapist, Vedic Chanting Teacher, Past President of Yoga Australia, Past Chair of IAYT Certification Committee, Past President of Yoga New Zealand, Australia.[1]

Rachel Krentzman, PT, E-RYT, C-IAYT, Physiotherapist, Yoga Therapist, Author and Hakomi Psychotherapist, Israel.[2]

Hansa Knox Johnson, C-IAYT, E-RYT-500, YACEP, KCYT, owner of PranaYoga and Āyurveda Mandala, USA.[3]

Swami Sivasankariananda, Director, Los Angeles Sivananda Yoga Vedanta Center, USA.[4]

Kari Ross-Berry, E-RYT-500, YACEP, C-IAYT, Associate Professor of Exercise Science: Yoga at Southwestern College, MA in Yoga Studies, MS in Exercise Science, USA.[5]

Susan Chapman®, MA, MFA, PGYT, C-IAYT, E-RYT-500, YTRx™-1000, POLY, YACEP, Yoga Therapist, Instructor, Scholar, and Coach, USA.[6]

---

1 https://yogainstitute.com.au/faculty-3/leanne-davis
2 https://happybackyoga.com
3 https://pyamandala.com/our-teachers
4 https://sivanandala.org
5 https://r.yogaalliance.org/TeacherPublicProfile/tid/20834
6 www.susanchapmanyoga.com

CHAPTER 8, THE GIFT OF YOGA

Michael Lee, MA, DipSocSci, C-IAYT, Founder of Phoenix Rising Yoga Therapy, USA.[7]

Joanne Wohlmuth, MA, E-RYT-500, YACEP, C-IAYT, Yoga Trainer/Instructor/OD Consultant at Yoga On The Rock, Bermuda.

Steffany Moonaz, PhD, C-IAYT, Professor and Research Director at Southern California University of Health Sciences, Founder/Director of Yoga for Arthritis, USA.[8]

Janet M. Caldwell, MS, C-IAYT, Healing Therapist, USA.

Amy Wheeler, PhD, C-IAYT, Founder of Optimal State Yoga Therapy School, USA.[9]

Susan Tebb, PhD, LSW, RYT-500, C-IAYT, USA.

CHAPTER 9, INNER GUIDANCE

Yogacharini Lee Majewski, MA, C-IAYT, C-IYA, Author and Founding Director of the Yoga for Health Institute, Canada.[10]

Stephen (Stoma) Parker, PsyD, Emeritus Psychologist, C-IAYT, E-RYT-500, YACEP, USA.

Durga Leela, BA, AP-NAMA, C-IAYT, eRYT Founder and Author of Yoga of Recovery, USA.[11]

Laurie Angress, C-IAYT, Certified Yoga Therapist, iRest Meditation Instructor, Seven Directions Breathwork Facilitator, USA.[12]

Lori Rubenstein Fazzio, DPT, PT, MAppSc, C-IAYT, Yoga Chikitsa Acharia,

---

7   https://usabp.org/PhoenixRisingYogaTherapy
8   https://integralyogatherapy.org/people/steffany-moonaz
9   https://amywheeler.com/iayt
10 www.yogaforhealth.institute
11 www.yogaofrecovery.com
12 www.mindfulyogatherapy.net/about-laurie

Clinical Professor of Yoga and Health, Loyola Marymount University Graduate Yoga Studies, Bellarmine College of Liberal Arts, USA.

Reverend Danielle Atkinson, OCT, C-IAYT, E-RYT-500, CAHP/CCA, Ayurvedic Professional, Canada.

SEEKING OUT

Anne Pitman, MSc, C-IAYT, Director of the School of Embodied Yoga Therapy, Associate Professor at the University of Ottawa, Co-Author of Yoga Therapy Across the Cancer Care Continuum, Canada.[13]

Marilyn Peppers-Citizen, PhD, MBA, NBC-HWC, E-RYT-500, C-IAYT, USA.[14]

Sat Bir Singh Khalsa, PhD, Corresponding Member of the Faculty of Medicine, Harvard Medical School, USA.[15]

Robert Butera, PhD, MDiv, PE, C-IAYT, Director of YogaLife Institute, Comprehensive Yoga Therapy, USA.[16]

Lisa Kaley-Isley, PhD, E-RYT-500, C-IAYT, Yoga Teacher, Yoga Therapist, Yoga Therapy Educator, USA.[17]

Gary Kraftsow, MA, E-RYT-500, C-IAYT, Founder/Director of American Viniyoga Institute, LC, USA.[18]

Stephanie Lopez, LISW-S, C-IAYT, President, iRest Institute, USA.[19]

---

13 https://thechi.ca/our-team/anne-pitman
14 www.arqat.org/marilyn-peppers-citizen
15 https://sleep.hms.harvard.edu/faculty-staff/sat-bir-singh-khalsa
16 www.yogalifeinstitute.com/teaching-team
17 https://lifetreeyoga.com/lisa-kaley-isley
18 www.viniyoga.com
19 https://shop.irest.org/pages/stephanie-lopez

CHAPTER 11, SPIRITUALITY IN ACTION

Helene Couvrette, C-IAYT, E-RYT-500, Yoga Educator, Founder/President H~OM Yoga School, Cofounder/President MISTY (Montreal International Symposium on Therapeutic Yoga), Canada.[20]

Richard Miller, PhD, F-IAYT, E-RYT-500, Founder of iRest Institute, Developer of IR-iRest, USA.[21]

Sri Vasudeva, International Spiritual Teacher, Trinidad & Tobago.[22]

Julie Rowland, C-IAYT, Certified Yoga Therapist, UCLA Health Integrative Medicine Collaborative, Ornish Lifestyle Medicine, Loyola Marymount University, Yoga Therapy Mentor, USA.[23]

Jivana Heyman, C-IAYT, E-RYT-500, Director, Accessible Yoga, USA.[24]

Yogacharya Dr. Ananda Balayogi Bhavanani, Ashram Acharya, ICYER-Ananda Ashram, Madathipathi, Sri Kambaliswamy Madam, Chairman and Mentor Yoganjali Natyalayam, Director and Professor of Yoga Therapy, Institute of Salutogenesis and Complementary Medicine, Sri Balaji Vidyapeeth, Pondicherry, India.[25]

---

20 www.homyogacenter.com/helenecouvrette-yogatherapist-yogateacher-yogatherapytrainingleadeducator
21 www.iRest.org
22 https://sri-vasudeva.com; www.blue-star.org
23 https://bethechangeyoga.com/project/julie-rowland-c-iayt-faculty
24 www.accessibleyogaschool.com
25 www.yogaiya.in/profile/ananda-balayogi-bhavanani

RAISING READERS
Books Build Bright Futures

Dear Reader,

We'd love your attention for one more page to tell you about the crisis in children's reading, and what we can all do.

Studies have shown that reading for fun is the **single biggest predictor of a child's future life chances** – more than family circumstance, parents' educational background or income. It improves academic results, mental health, wealth, communication skills, ambition and happiness.[1]

The number of children reading for fun is in rapid decline. Young people have a lot of competition for their time. In 2024, 1 in 10 children and young people in the UK aged 5 to 18 did not own a single book at home.[2]

Hachette works extensively with schools, libraries and literacy charities, but here are some ways we can all raise more readers:

- Reading to children for just 10 minutes a day makes a difference
- Don't give up if children aren't regular readers – there will be books for them!
- Visit bookshops and libraries to get recommendations
- Encourage them to listen to audiobooks
- Support school libraries
- Give books as gifts

There's a lot more information about how to encourage children to read on our website: **www.RaisingReaders.co.uk**

Thank you for reading.

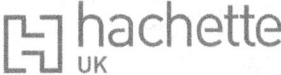

---

1 OECD, '21st-Century Readers: Developing Literacy Skills in a Digital World', 2021, https://www.oecd.org/en/publications/21st-century-readers_a83d84cb-en.html
2 National Literacy Trust, 'Book Ownership in 2024', November 2024, https://literacytrust.org.uk/research-services/research-reports/book-ownership-in-2024